CALORIE DIET FOOD LIST

The comprehensive guide to what food to avoid and eat with ingredient list for Obesity, Diabetes and Heart Disease

Jane Galaz

Table of Contents

Introduction...3

Understanding Caloric Intake.. 8

    What is a Calorie?... 8

    Importance of Caloric Balance... 12

    How to Calculate Your Daily Caloric Needs............................... 16

Part I: Foods to Eat... 20

Fruits and Vegetables.. 20

    Benefits of Fresh Produce.. 20

    Low-calorie Fruits.. 33

    Low-calorie Vegetables.. 34

    Whole Grains and Legumes... 45

    Lean Proteins.. 53

    Dairy and Alternatives... 63

Healthy Fats..73

　　Hydration.. 81

Part II: Foods to Avoid..88

　　Sugary Foods and Beverages.................................88

　　Refined Carbohydrates..97

　　Processed and Packaged Foods............................104

　　High Fat and Fried Foods.......................................109

　　High Calorie Condiments and Sauces....................115

Part III: Meal Planning and Recipes..........................127

　　Creating Balanced Meals.......................................127

　　Building a Low-calorie Plate.................................. 131

　　Portion Control Tips.. 135

　　Sample Meal Plans.. 139

　　7Day Low-calorie Meal Plan.................................. 142

　　Vegetarian and Vegan Options.............................. 146

Healthy Recipe Ideas.. 150

　　Breakfast... 150

　　Lunch... 154

Quinoa Salad with Veggies is a nutritious and delicious option for a calorie-conscious lunch...................................... 154

For this recipe, you'll need the following ingredients: 1 cup quinoa, 2 cups water, 1 cup cherry tomatoes (halved), 1 cucumber (diced), 1 bell pepper (diced), 1/4 cup red onion (finely chopped), 1/4 cup fresh parsley (chopped), 1/4 cup feta cheese (crumbled),

2 tablespoons olive oil, 1 tablespoon lemon juice, salt, and pepper to taste.. 154

To prepare the quinoa salad, start by rinsing the quinoa under cold water. In a medium saucepan, bring the quinoa and water to a boil. Reduce the heat to low, cover, and simmer for 15 minutes or until the water is absorbed and the quinoa is tender. Remove from heat and let it cool.. 154

In a large bowl, combine the cherry tomatoes, cucumber, bell pepper, red onion, parsley, and feta cheese. Add the cooled quinoa and mix well. In a small bowl, whisk together the olive oil, lemon juice, salt, and pepper. Pour the dressing over the salad and toss to combine.. 154

Nutritional information per serving includes 250 calories, 8g protein, 12g fat, 28g carbohydrates, and 4g fiber. The serving size is approximately 1 cup, and the total cooking time is about 25 minutes. This quinoa salad is a perfect balance of protein, healthy fats, and fiber, making it a satisfying and nutritious lunch option. 155

Grilled Chicken Wrap is another excellent choice for a healthy lunch. The ingredients required for this recipe are: 1 boneless, skinless chicken breast, 1 tablespoon olive oil, salt, pepper, 1/2 teaspoon paprika, 1/2 teaspoon garlic powder, 1 whole wheat tortilla, 1/2 avocado (sliced), 1/2 cup lettuce (shredded), 1/4 cup tomatoes (diced), and 2 tablespoons Greek yogurt.................155

To prepare the grilled chicken wrap, start by preheating the grill to medium-high heat. In a small bowl, mix the olive oil, salt, pepper, paprika, and garlic powder. Brush the chicken breast with the seasoned oil mixture. Grill the chicken for 6-7 minutes per side or until the internal temperature reaches 165°F.............. 155

Remove the chicken from the grill and let it rest for a few minutes before slicing it into strips. Warm the whole wheat tortilla in a dry skillet over medium heat for about 1 minute on each side. Lay the tortilla flat and spread the Greek yogurt in the center. Add the sliced chicken, avocado, lettuce, and tomatoes. Roll up the tortilla, tucking in the sides as you go 155

Nutritional information per serving includes 350 calories, 30g protein, 15g fat, 25g carbohydrates, and 7g fiber. The serving size is 1 wrap, and the total cooking time is approximately 20 minutes. This grilled chicken wrap is packed with protein and healthy fats, making it a filling and nutritious lunch option 156

Both of these lunch recipes are designed to be low in calories while providing essential nutrients to keep you satisfied and energized throughout the day. The quinoa salad with veggies offers a refreshing and light option, while the grilled chicken wrap provides a heartier and more substantial meal 156

By incorporating these recipes into your lunch rotation, you can enjoy delicious and healthy meals that align with your calorie-conscious diet goals 156

Dinner 157

Conclusion 162

Introduction

Emma had always been an adventurous soul. Her life was filled with hiking trips, spontaneous road trips, and latenight dance parties with friends. But lately, she found herself slowing down.

She was constantly tired, her energy levels plummeted, and she noticed that her favorite jeans no longer fit. One morning, after a particularly restless night, she stood in front of her mirror, taking in her reflection with a sigh.

"I need to make a change," she whispered to herself. Emma decided it was time to take control of her health and wellbeing. She knew she needed guidance, a structured plan that was easy to follow and would yield real results.

Chapter 2: Discovering the Guide

Emma spent hours researching online, sifting through endless articles and diet plans that promised quick fixes. She felt overwhelmed and frustrated. That evening, while chatting with her friend Lily over a cup of herbal tea, she poured out her frustrations.

"You know, I've been using this amazing guide called the 'Calorie Diet Food List'," Lily said, her eyes lighting up. "It's not just a diet; it's a complete lifestyle change. It helped me understand what foods to eat and which ones to avoid, all while staying within my calorie limits. I've never felt better!"

Intrigued, Emma asked Lily to tell her more. Lily explained how the guide was divided into easytofollow sections, detailing the benefits of various foods, meal planning tips, and even delicious recipes. The best part? It was simple to understand and incredibly motivating.

Chapter 3: A New Beginning

The next day, Emma purchased the "Calorie Diet Food List" guide. As she flipped through the pages, she felt a sense of hope and excitement. The introduction was welcoming and informative, explaining the importance of caloric intake and how to calculate her daily needs.

She learned about the benefits of fresh produce, whole grains, lean proteins, and healthy fats.
The guide also highlighted foods to avoid, such as sugary snacks, refined carbohydrates, and processed foods.

With each chapter, Emma felt more empowered. The guide didn't just tell her what to eat; it educated her on why certain foods were better for her body and how they contributed to her overall health. She was particularly impressed with the meal planning section, which provided practical tips for creating balanced meals and included sample meal plans for different dietary preferences.

Chapter 4: Putting Knowledge into Action

Emma decided to start her journey with a 7day meal plan suggested in the guide. She made a shopping list, filled her cart with vibrant fruits, crisp vegetables, lean meats, and wholesome grains. She felt a sense of accomplishment as she prepared her first meal: a colorful quinoa salad with fresh veggies and grilled chicken.

Throughout the week, Emma followed the guide religiously. She enjoyed smoothie bowls for breakfast, hearty salads for lunch, and delicious dinners like baked salmon with asparagus. She even found new favorite snacks, like Greek yogurt with berries and hummus with veggie sticks.

As the days passed, Emma noticed significant changes. Her energy levels soared, her sleep improved, and she felt more confident and positive. She no longer felt the need to snack mindlessly or reach for sugary treats. The "Calorie Diet Food List" had given her the tools to make healthier choices without feeling deprived.

Chapter 5: The Transformation

By the end of the month, Emma's transformation was evident. She had lost weight, her skin glowed, and she felt stronger and more vibrant than ever before. Her friends and family noticed the change and often asked her for her secret. Emma was more than happy to share her journey and recommend the guide that had helped her achieve such remarkable results.

One evening, as Emma relaxed on her couch with a cup of herbal tea, she reflected on her journey. The "Calorie Diet Food List" had not only helped her lose weight but had also taught her the value of balanced, nutritious eating.

She realized that her journey was just beginning and that the guide would continue to be her trusted companion on the path to lifelong health and wellness.

Conclusion: A Message to the Reader

Dear reader, if you find yourself feeling stuck, tired, or simply wanting to improve your health, I highly recommend the "Calorie Diet Food List." This guide is more than just a list of foods; it is a comprehensive resource that educates, motivates, and supports you every step of the way. Whether you're looking to lose weight, boost your energy, or simply make healthier choices, this guide will be your trusted ally.

Take the first step towards a healthier, happier you. Invest in the "Calorie Diet Food List" today and embark on a transformative journey just like Emma did. Your future self will thank you.

Understanding Caloric Intake

What is a Calorie?

A calorie is a unit of energy that is commonly used to quantify the energy content in food and beverages. It measures how much energy you get from consuming a particular food or drink, and this energy is essential for the body's various functions, from breathing and circulating blood to physical activity and maintaining body temperature.

When we talk about calories in the context of diet and nutrition, we're often referring to kilocalories (kcal), which are equal to 1,000 calories. For simplicity, we use the term calorie, but it's important to understand this distinction when reading nutritional information.

Understanding caloric intake is crucial for managing body weight and overall health. The body needs a certain number of calories each day to function properly, known as the Basal Metabolic Rate (BMR), which accounts for the energy expended at rest.
On top of that, additional calories are required to fuel physical activities and bodily processes such as digestion.

Consuming more calories than the body needs can lead to weight gain because the excess energy is stored as fat. Conversely, consuming fewer calories than needed can lead to weight loss as the body uses stored fat for energy.

The balance between calories consumed and calories burned is the key to weight management. This balance is influenced by several factors, including age, gender, weight, height, and activity level. For instance, an active young adult requires more calories than a sedentary older adult due to differences in metabolism and physical activity.

The Calorie Diet Food List helps individuals navigate their caloric needs by providing information on foods that are rich in essential nutrients yet low in calories, making it easier to maintain this balance.

When choosing foods from the Calorie Diet Food List, it's important to focus on nutrient-dense options. These are foods that provide a high amount of vitamins, minerals, and other beneficial compounds relative to their caloric content.

Examples include fruits, vegetables, lean proteins, whole grains, and healthy fats. Eating these foods ensures that your body gets the nutrients it needs without consuming excessive calories, which can help prevent weight gain and promote overall health.

One of the benefits of understanding caloric intake is the ability to make informed dietary choices. By being aware of the calorie content of different foods, you can better manage portion sizes and make healthier substitutions.

For example, swapping high-calorie, low-nutrient snacks like chips or cookies with low-calorie, nutrient-dense options like carrot sticks or a piece of fruit can significantly reduce your overall caloric intake while still providing satisfaction and essential nutrients.

In addition to managing weight, understanding caloric intake can also help improve energy levels and prevent chronic diseases.

Consuming the right amount of calories from nutritious foods supports optimal body function, boosts energy, and can reduce the risk of developing conditions such as heart disease, diabetes, and certain cancers.

The Calorie Diet Food List is a valuable resource in this regard, guiding you towards foods that support a healthy, balanced diet.

Ultimately, understanding calories and how they affect your body empowers you to take control of your health. By using the Calorie Diet Food List to make smart food choices, you can ensure that your diet provides the energy and nutrients your body needs while helping you achieve and maintain a healthy weight.

This knowledge is not just about counting calories but about making informed decisions that contribute to long-term well-being and vitality.

Importance of Caloric Balance

Caloric balance is a fundamental concept in the realm of nutrition and diet, playing a crucial role in maintaining overall health and achieving weight-related goals.

At its core, caloric balance refers to the equilibrium between the number of calories consumed through food and beverages and the number of calories expended through bodily functions and physical activities.

Understanding this balance is essential for anyone aiming to manage their weight, whether the goal is to lose, gain, or maintain it.

The human body requires a certain number of calories to perform basic physiological functions such as breathing, circulating blood, and cell production. This baseline caloric need is known as the Basal Metabolic Rate (BMR).

On top of BMR, additional calories are burned through physical activities, ranging from walking and household chores to vigorous exercise.

When the total caloric intake from food matches the total caloric expenditure, the body maintains its current weight. This state is known as being in caloric balance or energy balance.

Consuming more calories than the body uses leads to a caloric surplus. This surplus energy is stored in the body as fat, resulting in weight gain over time. On the other hand, consuming fewer calories than the body needs results in a caloric deficit.

To meet its energy requirements, the body then taps into stored fat, leading to weight loss. Thus, understanding caloric balance is pivotal for anyone looking to lose weight, as achieving a consistent caloric deficit is necessary to reduce body fat.

A well-structured calorie diet food list is an invaluable tool for managing caloric intake effectively. Such a list categorizes foods based on their caloric content and nutritional value, guiding individuals to make informed choices about what to eat.

By emphasizing low-calorie, nutrient-dense foods like fruits, vegetables, whole grains, and lean proteins, the diet plan helps create a caloric deficit without compromising on essential nutrients.

Conversely, it advises limiting or avoiding high-calorie, nutrient-poor foods like sugary snacks, refined grains, and processed foods, which can lead to caloric surplus and weight gain.

Adhering to a calorie diet food list also helps individuals develop a more mindful approach to eating. It encourages portion control and awareness of the caloric content of different foods, making it easier to balance meals throughout the day.

This mindfulness extends to recognizing the hidden calories in beverages and condiments, which can often be overlooked but contribute significantly to overall caloric intake. By being conscious of these details, individuals can better manage their energy balance and avoid unintentional weight gain.

Moreover, understanding caloric balance underscores the importance of physical activity in weight management. While diet plays a significant role in controlling caloric intake, regular exercise increases caloric expenditure, contributing to a caloric deficit necessary for weight loss.

Exercise also has numerous other health benefits, including improved cardiovascular health, stronger muscles and bones, and better mental well-being.

A calorie diet food list, paired with a consistent exercise routine, forms a comprehensive approach to achieving and maintaining a healthy weight.

Incorporating the principles of caloric balance into daily life involves not just short-term dietary changes but also long-term lifestyle adjustments. It requires commitment to a balanced diet, regular physical activity, and continuous self-monitoring of caloric intake and expenditure.

This holistic approach ensures that individuals not only reach their weight goals but also sustain them, fostering overall health and vitality.

Understanding and maintaining caloric balance is crucial for effective weight management and overall well-being. A well-planned calorie diet food list provides the necessary framework to make informed dietary choices, helping individuals achieve a harmonious balance between caloric intake and expenditure.

By integrating these principles into their lifestyle, individuals can enjoy the benefits of a healthier, more energetic, and fulfilling life.

How to Calculate Your Daily Caloric Needs

Calculating your daily caloric needs is a crucial step in achieving your health and fitness goals. Understanding how many calories your body requires to function optimally allows you to make informed dietary choices.

This process begins with determining your Basal Metabolic Rate (BMR), which is the number of calories your body needs to maintain basic physiological functions like breathing, circulation, and cell production while at rest. Various factors influence your BMR, including age, gender, weight, height, and body composition.

Online calculators can help estimate your BMR by inputting these details, providing a personalized starting point for your caloric needs.

Once you have your BMR, the next step is to consider your level of physical activity. The more active you are, the more calories your body requires to sustain your energy levels. To account for this, you multiply your BMR by an activity factor.

This factor varies depending on your lifestyle: sedentary (little to no exercise), lightly active (light exercise or sports 1-3 days a week), moderately active (moderate exercise or sports 3-5 days a week), very active (hard exercise or sports 6-7 days a week), or super active (very hard exercise, physical job, or training twice a day).

This calculation gives you your Total Daily Energy Expenditure (TDEE), which is the total number of calories you need to maintain your current weight.

For those looking to lose weight, creating a caloric deficit is essential. This means consuming fewer calories than your TDEE. A common and effective approach is to reduce your daily intake by 500-750 calories, which can result in a safe and sustainable weight loss of about 1-1.5 pounds per week.

However, it's crucial not to drop your calorie intake too low, as this can lead to nutrient deficiencies, muscle loss, and other health issues. Balancing your diet to ensure you receive adequate nutrition while in a caloric deficit is key to maintaining health and energy levels.

On the other hand, if your goal is to gain weight, you need to create a caloric surplus by consuming more calories than your TDEE. An increase of 250-500 calories per day is typically recommended to gain weight in a healthy and controlled manner. This should be paired with a balanced diet and regular strength training to promote muscle growth rather than fat accumulation.

Monitoring your progress and adjusting your caloric intake as needed will help you achieve your desired weight and body composition.

In addition to caloric intake, the quality of the calories consumed plays a significant role in achieving your health goals. The "Calorie Diet Food List" guide emphasizes the importance of choosing nutrient-dense foods that provide essential vitamins, minerals, and macronutrients.

Prioritizing whole foods such as fruits, vegetables, lean proteins, whole grains, and healthy fats ensures that your body receives the nutrients it needs to function efficiently and support your overall well-being.

Tracking your food intake can be immensely helpful in managing your caloric consumption.
Numerous apps and tools are available to help you log your meals and monitor your calorie intake. By keeping track of what you eat,

you can make adjustments as needed and stay on track with your dietary goals.

This practice also helps you become more mindful of portion sizes and the nutritional content of the foods you consume, making it easier to make healthier choices consistently.

Consistency and patience are vital when it comes to adjusting your caloric intake. Your body needs time to adapt to changes in diet and activity levels.

Regularly reassessing your caloric needs and making incremental adjustments based on your progress will ensure that you continue to move towards your goals effectively.

Remember, the "Calorie Diet Food List" guide is not just about counting calories but about fostering a healthy relationship with food and creating sustainable eating habits that support long-term health and wellness.

Part I: Foods to Eat

Fruits and Vegetables

Benefits of Fresh Produce

Fresh produce, encompassing a wide variety of fruits and vegetables, plays a pivotal role in a calorie diet food list due to its numerous health benefits and its natural alignment with calorie-conscious eating.

Fruits and vegetables are naturally low in calories yet rich in essential nutrients, making them an ideal choice for those seeking to manage their weight while maintaining a balanced diet. Their high water and fiber content contributes to a sense of fullness and satisfaction, reducing the likelihood of overeating and aiding in weight management efforts.

The vibrant array of vitamins, minerals, and antioxidants found in fresh produce supports overall health and well-being. Fruits and vegetables are abundant in vitamins A, C, and E, which are vital for immune function, skin health, and vision.

Additionally, minerals such as potassium, found in bananas and leafy greens, help regulate blood pressure and support cardiovascular health. Consuming a variety of colorful fruits and vegetables ensures that the body receives a wide spectrum of nutrients, which can enhance metabolic processes and energy levels.

Fiber is another crucial component of fresh produce that significantly benefits those following a calorie-controlled diet. Dietary fiber, present in high amounts in vegetables like broccoli, spinach, and carrots, promotes healthy digestion and regular bowel movements.

Fiber also slows the absorption of sugar into the bloodstream, preventing spikes in blood sugar levels and aiding in sustained energy throughout the day. This can be particularly beneficial for individuals aiming to avoid the energy crashes and cravings associated with refined and processed foods.

Fresh produce also offers an array of natural compounds that have been linked to disease prevention. Antioxidants, such as flavonoids, carotenoids, and polyphenols, are abundant in fruits and vegetables like berries, tomatoes, and bell peppers.

These compounds help neutralize free radicals, reducing oxidative stress and lowering the risk of chronic diseases such as heart disease, diabetes, and certain cancers. Incorporating a variety of fresh produce into the diet can therefore contribute to long-term health and longevity.

The versatility of fruits and vegetables makes them easy to incorporate into any meal plan. They can be enjoyed raw, steamed, roasted, or blended into smoothies, providing endless culinary possibilities while keeping meals interesting and satisfying.

This adaptability ensures that individuals on a calorie-controlled diet can enjoy a diverse range of flavors and textures, which can help sustain long-term adherence to healthy eating habits.

Moreover, fresh produce is naturally low in fats and sugars, making it a safe and effective choice for reducing overall caloric intake without compromising nutritional value. The natural sweetness of fruits like apples, oranges, and grapes can satisfy sweet cravings, reducing the reliance on high-calorie, sugary snacks and desserts.

Vegetables, on the other hand, can serve as the foundation of savory dishes, providing volume and nutrients without adding excessive calories.

Incorporating a generous amount of fresh fruits and vegetables into a calorie diet food list not only supports weight management and overall health but also fosters a positive relationship with food.

By focusing on the abundant, nutrient-rich options that nature provides, individuals can enjoy delicious and satisfying meals while nourishing their bodies and promoting optimal health.

The benefits of fresh produce are multifaceted, making them an indispensable component of any effective calorie-controlled diet plan.

Low-calorie Fruits

Here's a detailed table about low-calorie fruits in relation to a calorie diet food list, including ingredients, instructions, nutritional information, serving size, and cooking time:

Notes:

- **Preparation Time:** All fruits can be prepared within 5-10 minutes.
- **Serving Suggestions:** Enjoy these fruits as snacks, in fruit salads, or as part of breakfast.
- **Nutritional Benefits:** These low-calorie fruits are rich in vitamins, minerals, and fiber, making them excellent choices for a calorie-conscious diet. They provide essential nutrients while keeping the calorie intake low, aiding in weight management and overall health.

Fruit	Ingredients	Instructions	Nutritional Information (per serving)	Serving Size	Cooking Time
Strawberries	1 cup strawberries	Wash and slice the strawberries.	50 calories, 1g protein, 0.5g fat, 12g carbohydrates, 3g fiber, 89mg vitamin C	1 cup	None
Watermelon	1 cup watermelon cubes	Cut watermelon into cubes.	46 calories, 0.9g protein, 0.2g fat, 11.5g carbohydrates, 0.6g	1 cup	None

Fruit	Ingredients	Instructions	Nutritional Information (per serving)	Serving Size	Cooking Time
			fiber, 12.3mg vitamin C		
Grapefruit	1 medium grapefruit	Peel and segment the grapefruit.	52 calories, 1g protein, 0.2g fat, 13g carbohydrates, 2g fiber, 38mg vitamin C	1 medium	None
Cantaloupe	1 cup cantaloupe cubes	Cut cantaloupe into cubes.	53 calories, 1.3g protein, 0.3g fat,	1 cup	None

Fruit	Ingredients	Instructions	Nutritional Information (per serving)	Serving Size	Cooking Time
			13g carbohydrates, 1.4g fiber, 57mg vitamin C		
Papaya	1 cup papaya cubes	Peel and cut papaya into cubes.	55 calories, 0.9g protein, 0.2g fat, 14g carbohydrates, 2.5g fiber, 88.3mg vitamin C	1 cup	None

Fruit	Ingredients	Instructions	Nutritional Information (per serving)	Serving Size	Cooking Time
Peach	1 medium peach	Wash and slice the peach.	59 calories, 1.4g protein, 0.4g fat, 14.5g carbohydrates, 2.3g fiber, 10mg vitamin C	1 medium	None
Orange	1 medium orange	Peel and segment the orange.	62 calories, 1.2g protein, 0.2g fat, 15.4g carbohydrates, 3.1g	1 medium	None

Fruit	Ingredients	Instructions	Nutritional Information (per serving)	Serving Size	Cooking Time
			fiber, 70mg vitamin C		
Blueberries	1 cup blueberries	Wash the blueberries.	84 calories, 1.1g protein, 0.5g fat, 21g carbohydrates, 3.6g fiber, 14.4mg vitamin C	1 cup	None
Apples	1 medium apple	Wash and slice the apple.	95 calories, 0.5g protein, 0.3g fat,	1 medium	None

Fruit	Ingredients	Instructions	Nutritional Information (per serving)	Serving Size	Cooking Time
			25g carbohydrates, 4.4g fiber, 8.4mg vitamin C		
Raspberries	1 cup raspberries	Wash the raspberries.	64 calories, 1.5g protein, 0.8g fat, 15g carbohydrates, 8g fiber, 32.2mg vitamin C	1 cup	None

Fruit	Ingredients	Instructions	Nutritional Information (per serving)	Serving Size	Cooking Time
Kiwi	2 medium kiwis	Peel and slice the kiwis.	90 calories, 2g protein, 0.9g fat, 22g carbohydrates, 4.3g fiber, 137.2mg vitamin C	2 medium	None
Pineapple	1 cup pineapple chunks	Peel and cut pineapple into chunks.	82 calories, 0.9g protein, 0.2g fat, 21.7g carbohydrates, 2.3g	1 cup	None

Fruit	Ingredients	Instructions	Nutritional Information (per serving)	Serving Size	Cooking Time
			fiber, 78.9mg vitamin C		
Cherries	1 cup cherries	Wash and pit the cherries.	97 calories, 1.6g protein, 0.3g fat, 25g carbohydrates, 3.2g fiber, 10.8mg vitamin C	1 cup	None
Mango	1 cup mango slices	Peel and slice the mango.	99 calories, 1.4g protein, 0.6g fat,	1 cup	None

Fruit	Ingredients	Instructions	Nutritional Information (per serving)	Serving Size	Cooking Time
			25g carbohydrates, 2.6g fiber, 60.1mg vitamin C		
Plum	1 medium plum	Wash and slice the plum.	30 calories, 0.5g protein, 0.2g fat, 7.5g carbohydrates, 0.9g fiber, 6.3mg vitamin C	1 medium	None

Low-calorie Vegetables

Sure! Here's a comprehensive table detailing 15 low-calorie vegetables, including their ingredients, instructions, nutritional information, serving size, and cooking time:

Vegetable	Ingredients	Instructions	Nutritional Information (per serving)	Serving Size	Cooking Time
Spinach	Fresh spinach	1. Rinse spinach leaves thoroughly. 2. Steam for 2-3 minutes until wilted.	Calories: 7 Protein: 1g Carbs: 1g Fiber: 1g Fat: 0g	1 cup	2-3 minutes
Lettuce	Fresh lettuce	1. Wash and chop lettuce. 2. Use raw	Calories: 5 Protein: 0.5g Carbs: 1g	1 cup	No cooking

Vegetable	Ingredients	Instructions	Nutritional Information (per serving)	Serving Size	Cooking Time
		in salads or sandwiches.	Fiber: 1g Fat: 0g		required
Cucumber	Fresh cucumber	1. Wash cucumber. 2. Slice or dice as desired. 3. Use raw in salads or as a snack.	Calories: 8 Protein: 0.3g Carbs: 2g Fiber: 0.3g Fat: 0g	1/2 cup	No cooking required
Zucchini	Fresh zucchini	1. Wash and slice zucchini. 2. Sauté in a	Calories: 19 Protein: 1.5g Carbs: 4g	1 cup	5-7 minutes

Vegetable	Ingredients	Instructions	Nutritional Information (per serving)	Serving Size	Cooking Time
		non-stick pan for 5-7 minutes until tender.	Fiber: 1g Fat: 0g		
Bell Peppers	Fresh bell peppers	1. Wash and slice bell peppers. 2. Sauté or eat raw.	Calories: 24 Protein: 1g Carbs: 6g Fiber: 2g Fat: 0g	1/2 cup	5-7 minutes (if cooked)
Tomatoes	Fresh tomatoes	1. Wash and chop tomatoes. 2. Use raw in salads or	Calories: 22 Protein: 1g Carbs: 5g Fiber:	1/2 cup	Varies

Vegetable	Ingredients	Instructions	Nutritional Information (per serving)	Serving Size	Cooking Time
		cook in recipes.	1.5g Fat: 0.2g		
Carrots	Fresh carrots	1. Wash and peel carrots. 2. Slice or dice. 3. Eat raw or steam for 5-7 minutes.	Calories: 25 Protein: 0.5g Carbs: 6g Fiber: 2g Fat: 0g	1/2 cup	5-7 minutes
Broccoli	Fresh broccoli	1. Wash and chop broccoli. 2. Steam for 5-7 minutes until tender.	Calories: 31 Protein: 2.5g Carbs: 6g Fiber: 2.5g Fat: 0.3g	1 cup	5-7 minutes

Vegetable	Ingredients	Instructions	Nutritional Information (per serving)	Serving Size	Cooking Time
Cauliflower	Fresh cauliflower	1. Wash and chop cauliflower. 2. Steam for 5-7 minutes until tender.	Calories: 25 Protein: 2g Carbs: 5g Fiber: 2g Fat: 0.1g	1 cup	5-7 minutes
Celery	Fresh celery	1. Wash and chop celery. 2. Eat raw or add to salads and soups.	Calories: 6 Protein: 0.3g Carbs: 1.2g Fiber: 0.6g Fat: 0g	1/2 cup	No cooking required

Vegetable	Ingredients	Instructions	Nutritional Information (per serving)	Serving Size	Cooking Time
Kale	Fresh kale	1. Rinse kale leaves thoroughly. 2. Steam for 3-5 minutes until tender.	Calories: 33 Protein: 2.5g Carbs: 7g Fiber: 1.3g Fat: 0.5g	1 cup	3-5 minutes
Asparagus	Fresh asparagus	1. Rinse and trim asparagus. 2. Steam or sauté for 5-7 minutes until tender.	Calories: 20 Protein: 2g Carbs: 4g Fiber: 2g Fat: 0.2g	1/2 cup	5-7 minutes

Vegetable	Ingredients	Instructions	Nutritional Information (per serving)	Serving Size	Cooking Time
Green Beans	Fresh green beans	1. Wash and trim green beans. 2. Steam for 5-7 minutes until tender.	Calories: 17 Protein: 1g Carbs: 4g Fiber: 1.8g Fat: 0g	1/2 cup	5-7 minutes
Brussels Sprouts	Fresh Brussels sprouts	1. Rinse and trim Brussels sprouts. 2. Steam or roast for 15-20 minutes until tender.	Calories: 38 Protein: 3g Carbs: 8g Fiber: 3g Fat: 0.5g	1 cup	15-20 minutes

Vegetable	Ingredients	Instructions	Nutritional Information (per serving)	Serving Size	Cooking Time
Radishes	Fresh radishes	1. Wash and slice radishes. 2. Eat raw or add to salads.	Calories: 9 Protein: 0.4g Carbs: 2g Fiber: 1g Fat: 0g	1/2 cup	No cooking required

Tips for Incorporating Low-Calorie Vegetables into Your Diet:

- **Salads**: Create colorful and nutritious salads by mixing a variety of low-calorie vegetables.
- **Snacks**: Use raw vegetables like cucumber, celery, and carrots as crunchy, low-calorie snacks.
- **Side Dishes**: Steam or sauté vegetables like broccoli, cauliflower, and asparagus as healthy side dishes for your meals.
- **Soups and Stews**: Add chopped vegetables like tomatoes, carrots, and green beans to soups and stews for added nutrition and flavor.

Benefits of Low-Calorie Vegetables:

- **Weight Management**: Low-calorie vegetables are high in fiber and water content, which helps you feel full longer, reducing overall calorie intake.
- **Nutrient-Dense**: These vegetables are rich in essential vitamins, minerals, and antioxidants, promoting overall health.
- **Versatility**: They can be incorporated into a variety of dishes, making it easy to maintain a balanced diet.

Whole Grains and Legumes

When creating a calorie-conscious diet, incorporating whole grains and legumes can be both nutritious and satisfying. These food groups provide essential nutrients, fiber, and protein, making them ideal for maintaining energy levels and overall health.

Below is a detailed table listing 15 whole grains and legumes, including their ingredients, instructions, nutritional information, serving sizes, and cooking times.

Ingredient	Instructions	Nutritional Information (per serving)	Serving Size	Cooking Time
Quinoa	Rinse 1 cup quinoa. Boil 2 cups water, add quinoa, reduce heat, simmer for 15 mins.	222 calories, 4g fat, 39g carbs, 8g protein, 5g fiber	1 cup cooked	15 minutes
Brown Rice	Rinse 1 cup rice. Boil 2.5 cups water, add rice, reduce heat, simmer for 45 mins.	216 calories, 1.8g fat, 45g carbs, 5g protein, 3.5g fiber	1 cup cooked	45 minutes

Ingredient	Instructions	Nutritional Information (per serving)	Serving Size	Cooking Time
Farro	Rinse 1 cup farro. Boil 3 cups water, add farro, simmer for 30 mins. Drain excess water.	170 calories, 1g fat, 34g carbs, 7g protein, 5g fiber	1 cup cooked	30 minutes
Barley	Rinse 1 cup barley. Boil 3 cups water, add barley, reduce heat, simmer for 45 mins.	193 calories, 1g fat, 44g carbs, 4g protein, 6g fiber	1 cup cooked	45 minutes
Bulgur	Boil 1.5 cups water, add 1 cup	151 calories, 0.4g fat, 34g carbs, 5.6g	1 cup cooked	10 minutes

Ingredient	Instructions	Nutritional Information (per serving)	Serving Size	Cooking Time
	bulgur, cover, let sit for 10 mins, fluff with fork.	protein, 8g fiber		
Millet	Toast 1 cup millet in dry pan, boil 2.5 cups water, add millet, simmer for 20 mins.	207 calories, 1.7g fat, 41g carbs, 6g protein, 2.3g fiber	1 cup cooked	20 minutes
Oats	Boil 1 cup water, add 1/2 cup oats, simmer for 5 mins, stir occasionally.	154 calories, 3g fat, 27g carbs, 6g protein, 4g fiber	1 cup cooked	5 minutes

Ingredient	Instructions	Nutritional Information (per serving)	Serving Size	Cooking Time
Buckwheat	Rinse 1 cup buckwheat. Boil 2 cups water, add buckwheat, simmer for 20 mins.	155 calories, 1g fat, 33g carbs, 5.7g protein, 4.5g fiber	1 cup cooked	20 minutes
Spelt	Rinse 1 cup spelt. Boil 3 cups water, add spelt, simmer for 60 mins.	246 calories, 1.5g fat, 51g carbs, 10.6g protein, 7.5g fiber	1 cup cooked	60 minutes
Lentils	Rinse 1 cup lentils. Boil 2.5 cups water, add lentils, simmer for 25 mins.	230 calories, 0.8g fat, 39.9g carbs, 17.9g protein, 15.6g fiber	1 cup cooked	25 minutes

Ingredient	Instructions	Nutritional Information (per serving)	Serving Size	Cooking Time
Chickpeas	Soak 1 cup chickpeas overnight. Boil in fresh water for 1-2 hours until tender.	269 calories, 4.2g fat, 45g carbs, 14.5g protein, 12.5g fiber	1 cup cooked	60-120 minutes
Black Beans	Rinse 1 cup black beans. Boil 3 cups water, add beans, simmer for 1-2 hours until tender.	227 calories, 0.9g fat, 40.8g carbs, 15.2g protein, 15g fiber	1 cup cooked	60-120 minutes
Kidney Beans	Rinse 1 cup kidney beans. Boil 3 cups water, add	225 calories, 0.9g fat, 40.4g carbs, 15.4g	1 cup cooked	60-120 minutes

Ingredient	Instructions	Nutritional Information (per serving)	Serving Size	Cooking Time
	beans, simmer for 1-2 hours until tender.	protein, 13.6g fiber		
Navy Beans	Rinse 1 cup navy beans. Boil 3 cups water, add beans, simmer for 1-2 hours until tender.	255 calories, 1.1g fat, 47.3g carbs, 15g protein, 19.1g fiber	1 cup cooked	60-120 minutes
Green Peas	Boil 1 cup green peas for 3-5 mins until tender.	118 calories, 0.6g fat, 21g carbs, 8g protein, 7g fiber	1 cup cooked	3-5 minutes

Summary of Nutritional Benefits

Whole grains and legumes are essential components of a balanced, calorie-conscious diet. They provide a variety of nutrients such as:

- **Fiber**: Helps in digestion and maintaining a healthy weight.
- **Protein**: Crucial for muscle repair and overall body functions.
- **Vitamins and Minerals**: Whole grains and legumes are rich in B vitamins, iron, magnesium, and zinc.

Tips for Incorporating Whole Grains and Legumes into Your Diet

1. **Breakfast**: Start your day with a hearty bowl of oats or quinoa porridge.
2. **Lunch**: Include a serving of lentil or chickpea salad.
3. **Dinner**: Use brown rice or barley as a base for stir-fries and casseroles.
4. **Snacks**: Enjoy roasted chickpeas or spelt crackers as a nutritious snack.

By integrating these whole grains and legumes into your meals, you can enjoy a variety of flavors while maintaining a healthy, balanced diet that supports your calorie goals.

Lean Proteins

Here's a detailed, comprehensive content on "Lean Proteins" related to a calorie diet food list, including 15 lean protein ingredients.

Each entry includes the ingredient, instructions for preparation, nutritional information, serving size, and cooking time, all presented in a table format.

Ingredient	Instructions	Nutritional Information	Serving Size	Cooking Time
Chicken Breast	Season with salt, pepper, and herbs. Grill on medium heat for 6-7 minutes per side until internal temperature reaches 165°F.	165 calories, 31g protein, 3.6g fat per 4 oz serving	4 oz	12-14 minutes
Turkey Breast	Marinate in lemon juice and garlic. Bake at	135 calories, 30g protein, 1g fat per 4 oz serving	4 oz	20-25 minutes

Ingredient	Instructions	Nutritional Information	Serving Size	Cooking Time
	350°F for 20-25 minutes until internal temperature reaches 165°F.			
Salmon	Rub with olive oil, salt, and pepper. Bake at 375°F for 12-15 minutes until fish flakes easily with a fork.	206 calories, 22g protein, 13g fat per 4 oz serving	4 oz	12-15 minutes
Tuna	Season with soy sauce and ginger. Sear on high heat for 2-3 minutes per side until desired doneness.	145 calories, 25g protein, 4.9g fat per 4 oz serving	4 oz	4-6 minutes

Ingredient	Instructions	Nutritional Information	Serving Size	Cooking Time
Cod	Coat with a mixture of breadcrumbs and spices. Bake at 400°F for 10-12 minutes until fish flakes easily.	93 calories, 20g protein, 0.9g fat per 4 oz serving	4 oz	10-12 minutes
Egg Whites	Whisk with a pinch of salt. Cook in a non-stick pan over medium heat for 3-5 minutes, stirring occasionally.	17 calories, 3.6g protein, 0g fat per 1 large egg white	3 egg whites	3-5 minutes
Greek Yogurt	Enjoy plain or mix with fresh fruit and a drizzle of honey.	100 calories, 10g protein, 0g fat per 5.3 oz serving	5.3 oz	No cooking needed

Ingredient	Instructions	Nutritional Information	Serving Size	Cooking Time
Cottage Cheese	Serve with sliced tomatoes and a sprinkle of black pepper.	98 calories, 11g protein, 4.3g fat per 4 oz serving	4 oz	No cooking needed
Lean Beef	Season with salt and pepper. Grill or broil for 4-5 minutes per side for medium-rare, longer for more doneness.	150 calories, 24g protein, 4g fat per 4 oz serving	4 oz	8-10 minutes
Pork Tenderloin	Marinate in a mixture of olive oil, garlic, and rosemary. Roast at 400°F for 20-25	143 calories, 24g protein, 3.5g fat per 4 oz serving	4 oz	20-25 minutes

Ingredient	Instructions	Nutritional Information	Serving Size	Cooking Time
	minutes until internal temperature reaches 145°F.			
Tofu	Press to remove excess water, then cut into cubes. Stir-fry with vegetables and soy sauce over medium-high heat for 5-7 minutes.	94 calories, 10g protein, 5g fat per 4 oz serving	4 oz	5-7 minutes
Tempeh	Slice and marinate in soy sauce and spices. Sauté over medium heat for 4-5	160 calories, 15g protein, 9g fat per 4 oz serving	4 oz	8-10 minutes

Ingredient	Instructions	Nutritional Information	Serving Size	Cooking Time
	minutes per side.			
Shrimp	Season with Old Bay or similar seasoning. Sauté in a hot pan with olive oil for 2-3 minutes per side until pink and opaque.	84 calories, 18g protein, 1g fat per 4 oz serving	4 oz	4-6 minutes
Lentils	Rinse and boil in water with a pinch of salt for 20-25 minutes until tender. Drain and season with herbs.	113 calories, 9g protein, 0.4g fat per 1 cup cooked	1 cup	20-25 minutes

Ingredient	Instructions	Nutritional Information	Serving Size	Cooking Time
Black Beans	Rinse and boil with a bay leaf and a pinch of salt for 60-90 minutes until tender. Drain and season with cumin and lime juice.	227 calories, 15g protein, 0.9g fat per 1 cup cooked	1 cup	60-90 minutes

Summary:

This table provides a comprehensive guide to 15 lean proteins suitable for a calorie-conscious diet. Each protein source includes preparation instructions, nutritional information, serving size, and cooking time.

The proteins range from various meats like chicken, turkey, and lean beef to seafood such as salmon and shrimp, as well as vegetarian options like tofu, tempeh, and lentils. These lean proteins can help maintain muscle mass, support weight loss, and provide essential nutrients while keeping calorie intake in check.

Dairy and Alternatives

Here's a detailed, comprehensive content on "Lean Proteins" related to a calorie diet food list, including 15 lean protein ingredients. Each entry includes the ingredient, instructions for preparation, nutritional information, serving size, and cooking time, all presented in a table format.

Ingredient	Instructions	Nutritional Information	Serving Size	Cooking Time
Chicken Breast	Season with salt, pepper, and herbs. Grill on medium heat for 6-7 minutes per side until internal temperature reaches 165°F.	165 calories, 31g protein, 3.6g fat per 4 oz serving	4 oz	12-14 minutes
Turkey Breast	Marinate in lemon juice and garlic.	135 calories, 30g protein,	4 oz	20-25 minutes

Ingredient	Instructions	Nutritional Information	Serving Size	Cooking Time
	Bake at 350°F for 20-25 minutes until internal temperature reaches 165°F.	1g fat per 4 oz serving		
Salmon	Rub with olive oil, salt, and pepper. Bake at 375°F for 12-15 minutes until fish flakes easily with a fork.	206 calories, 22g protein, 13g fat per 4 oz serving	4 oz	12-15 minutes
Tuna	Season with soy sauce and ginger. Sear on high heat for 2-3 minutes per side until desired doneness.	145 calories, 25g protein, 4.9g fat per 4 oz serving	4 oz	4-6 minutes

Ingredient	Instructions	Nutritional Information	Serving Size	Cooking Time
Cod	Coat with a mixture of breadcrumbs and spices. Bake at 400°F for 10-12 minutes until fish flakes easily.	93 calories, 20g protein, 0.9g fat per 4 oz serving	4 oz	10-12 minutes
Egg Whites	Whisk with a pinch of salt. Cook in a non-stick pan over medium heat for 3-5 minutes, stirring occasionally.	17 calories, 3.6g protein, 0g fat per 1 large egg white	3 egg whites	3-5 minutes
Greek Yogurt	Enjoy plain or mix with fresh fruit and a	100 calories, 10g protein, 0g fat per 5.3 oz serving	5.3 oz	No cooking needed

Ingredient	Instructions	Nutritional Information	Serving Size	Cooking Time
	drizzle of honey.			
Cottage Cheese	Serve with sliced tomatoes and a sprinkle of black pepper.	98 calories, 11g protein, 4.3g fat per 4 oz serving	4 oz	No cooking needed
Lean Beef	Season with salt and pepper. Grill or broil for 4-5 minutes per side for medium-rare, longer for more doneness.	150 calories, 24g protein, 4g fat per 4 oz serving	4 oz	8-10 minutes
Pork Tenderloin	Marinate in a mixture of olive oil, garlic, and rosemary. Roast at 400°F	143 calories, 24g protein, 3.5g fat per 4 oz serving	4 oz	20-25 minutes

Ingredient	Instructions	Nutritional Information	Serving Size	Cooking Time
	for 20-25 minutes until internal temperature reaches 145°F.			
Tofu	Press to remove excess water, then cut into cubes. Stir-fry with vegetables and soy sauce over medium-high heat for 5-7 minutes.	94 calories, 10g protein, 5g fat per 4 oz serving	4 oz	5-7 minutes
Tempeh	Slice and marinate in soy sauce and spices. Sauté over medium heat for 4-5	160 calories, 15g protein, 9g fat per 4 oz serving	4 oz	8-10 minutes

Ingredient	Instructions	Nutritional Information	Serving Size	Cooking Time
	minutes per side.			
Shrimp	Season with Old Bay or similar seasoning. Sauté in a hot pan with olive oil for 2-3 minutes per side until pink and opaque.	84 calories, 18g protein, 1g fat per 4 oz serving	4 oz	4-6 minutes
Lentils	Rinse and boil in water with a pinch of salt for 20-25 minutes until tender. Drain and season with herbs.	113 calories, 9g protein, 0.4g fat per 1 cup cooked	1 cup	20-25 minutes

Ingredient	Instructions	Nutritional Information	Serving Size	Cooking Time
Black Beans	Rinse and boil with a bay leaf and a pinch of salt for 60-90 minutes until tender. Drain and season with cumin and lime juice.	227 calories, 15g protein, 0.9g fat per 1 cup cooked	1 cup	60-90 minutes

Summary:

This table provides a comprehensive guide to 15 lean proteins suitable for a calorie-conscious diet. Each protein source includes preparation instructions, nutritional information, serving size, and cooking time.

The proteins range from various meats like chicken, turkey, and lean beef to seafood such as salmon and shrimp, as well as vegetarian options like tofu, tempeh, and lentils. These lean proteins can help maintain muscle mass, support weight loss, and provide essential nutrients while keeping calorie intake in check.

Healthy Fats

Here's a detailed, comprehensive content on "Healthy Fats" related to a calorie diet food list, including 15 healthy fat ingredients.

Each entry includes the ingredient, instructions for preparation, nutritional information, serving size, and cooking time, all presented in a table format.

Ingredient	Instructions	Nutritional Information	Serving Size	Cooking Time
Avocado	Slice and add to salads, sandwiches, or toast. Sprinkle with a pinch of salt and a squeeze of lemon juice.	234 calories, 3g protein, 21g fat per 1 medium avocado	1 medium	No cooking needed
Olive Oil	Use as a dressing for salads or for sautéing vegetables. Drizzle over roasted dishes for extra flavor.	119 calories, 0g protein, 14g fat per 1 tablespoon	1 tablespoon	No cooking needed

Ingredient	Instructions	Nutritional Information	Serving Size	Cooking Time
Nuts (Almonds)	Eat as a snack, or chop and add to oatmeal, yogurt, or salads.	161 calories, 6g protein, 14g fat per 1 oz serving	1 oz	No cooking needed
Seeds (Chia)	Mix into smoothies, yogurt, or oatmeal. Soak in water or milk to make chia pudding.	138 calories, 4.7g protein, 8.7g fat per 1 oz serving	1 oz	No cooking needed
Coconut Oil	Use for sautéing vegetables or as a substitute for butter in baking.	121 calories, 0g protein, 14g fat per 1 tablespoon	1 tablespoon	No cooking needed

Ingredient	Instructions	Nutritional Information	Serving Size	Cooking Time
Nut Butter (Peanut)	Spread on toast, add to smoothies, or use as a dip for fruits and vegetables.	188 calories, 8g protein, 16g fat per 2 tablespoons	2 tablespoons	No cooking needed
Fatty Fish (Mackerel)	Season with salt, pepper, and herbs. Grill or bake at 375°F for 15-20 minutes until the fish flakes easily with a fork.	205 calories, 18g protein, 14g fat per 3 oz serving	3 oz	15-20 minutes
Dark Chocolate	Enjoy a few squares as a snack or dessert. Choose	155 calories, 2g protein, 12g fat per 1 oz serving	1 oz	No cooking needed

Ingredient	Instructions	Nutritional Information	Serving Size	Cooking Time
	dark chocolate with at least 70% cocoa content.			
Flaxseeds	Add to smoothies, yogurt, or baked goods. Grind them for better nutrient absorption.	150 calories, 5.2g protein, 11.8g fat per 2 tablespoons	2 tablespoons	No cooking needed
Eggs	Boil, scramble, or poach for a nutritious meal. Season with salt and pepper.	78 calories, 6g protein, 5g fat per 1 large egg	1 large egg	5-10 minutes (varies)

Ingredient	Instructions	Nutritional Information	Serving Size	Cooking Time
Cheese (Cheddar)	Eat as a snack, or add to sandwiches, salads, or omelets.	113 calories, 7g protein, 9g fat per 1 oz serving	1 oz	No cooking needed
Sunflower Seeds	Eat as a snack, or sprinkle on salads, yogurt, or oatmeal.	165 calories, 5.5g protein, 14g fat per 1 oz serving	1 oz	No cooking needed
Hemp Seeds	Add to smoothies, salads, or yogurt for a nutritional boost.	166 calories, 9.5g protein, 14.6g fat per 3 tablespoons	3 tablespoons	No cooking needed
Pumpkin Seeds	Eat as a snack, or add to salads, granola, or baked goods.	151 calories, 7g protein, 13g fat per 1 oz serving	1 oz	No cooking needed

Ingredient	Instructions	Nutritional Information	Serving Size	Cooking Time
Walnuts	Eat as a snack, or chop and add to oatmeal, yogurt, or salads.	185 calories, 4.3g protein, 18.5g fat per 1 oz serving	1 oz	No cooking needed

Summary:

This table provides a comprehensive guide to 15 healthy fats suitable for a calorie-conscious diet. Each fat source includes preparation instructions, nutritional information, serving size, and cooking time.

The fats range from plant-based options like avocados, nuts, and seeds to animal-based options like fatty fish and eggs. These healthy fats can help maintain overall health, support brain function, and provide essential fatty acids while keeping calorie intake in check.

Hydration

Here's a detailed, comprehensive content on "Hydration" related to a calorie diet food list, including 15 hydration ingredients.

Each entry includes the ingredient, instructions for preparation, nutritional information, serving size, and cooking time, all presented in a table format.

Ingredient	Instructions	Nutritional Information	Serving Size	Cooking Time
Cucumber	Slice and serve with a sprinkle of salt and lemon juice.	16 calories, 0.7g protein, 0.2g fat, 95% water per 1 cup slices	1 cup slices	No cooking needed
Watermelon	Cut into cubes and serve chilled.	46 calories, 0.9g protein, 0.2g fat, 92% water per 1 cup	1 cup	No cooking needed

Ingredient	Instructions	Nutritional Information	Serving Size	Cooking Time
Celery	Cut into sticks and serve with hummus.	16 calories, 0.8g protein, 0.2g fat, 95% water per 1 cup	1 cup	No cooking needed
Tomatoes	Slice and serve with a drizzle of olive oil and balsamic vinegar.	22 calories, 1.1g protein, 0.2g fat, 94% water per medium tomato	1 medium tomato	No cooking needed
Oranges	Peel and separate into segments.	62 calories, 1.2g protein, 0.2g fat, 86% water per medium orange	1 medium orange	No cooking needed

Ingredient	Instructions	Nutritional Information	Serving Size	Cooking Time
Strawberries	Wash and slice, serve with a sprinkle of sugar or honey.	49 calories, 1g protein, 0.5g fat, 91% water per 1 cup halves	1 cup halves	No cooking needed
Lettuce	Chop and serve as a base for salads.	5 calories, 0.5g protein, 0.1g fat, 96% water per 1 cup shredded	1 cup shredded	No cooking needed
Zucchini	Slice and sauté with olive oil and garlic for 5-7 minutes.	21 calories, 1.5g protein, 0.4g fat, 94% water per 1 cup sliced	1 cup sliced	5-7 minutes

Ingredient	Instructions	Nutritional Information	Serving Size	Cooking Time
Cantaloupe	Cut into cubes and serve chilled.	60 calories, 1.5g protein, 0.3g fat, 90% water per 1 cup cubes	1 cup cubes	No cooking needed
Peppers	Slice and serve with a dip or in salads.	31 calories, 1g protein, 0.2g fat, 92% water per 1 cup sliced	1 cup sliced	No cooking needed
Pineapple	Cut into chunks and serve fresh or grilled.	82 calories, 0.9g protein, 0.2g fat, 86% water per 1 cup chunks	1 cup chunks	No cooking needed

Ingredient	Instructions	Nutritional Information	Serving Size	Cooking Time
Grapefruit	Cut in half and scoop out segments, or peel and separate.	52 calories, 1g protein, 0.2g fat, 88% water per half medium grapefruit	Half grapefruit	No cooking needed
Spinach	Rinse and serve as a base for salads or sauté with garlic for 3-4 minutes.	7 calories, 0.9g protein, 0.1g fat, 91% water per 1 cup raw	1 cup raw	3-4 minutes (if sautéed)
Blueberries	Rinse and serve fresh, add to yogurt or oatmeal.	84 calories, 1.1g protein, 0.5g fat, 85% water per 1 cup	1 cup	No cooking needed

Ingredient	Instructions	Nutritional Information	Serving Size	Cooking Time
Bell Peppers	Slice and serve fresh, or roast at 400°F for 20 minutes.	24 calories, 1g protein, 0.2g fat, 92% water per 1 cup sliced	1 cup sliced	20 minutes (if roasted)

Summary:

This table provides a comprehensive guide to 15 hydration ingredients suitable for a calorie-conscious diet. Each ingredient includes preparation instructions, nutritional information, serving size, and cooking time.

These hydration-rich foods, ranging from fruits like watermelon, strawberries, and oranges to vegetables like cucumber, lettuce, and bell peppers, are perfect for maintaining proper hydration levels. They are high in water content and low in calories, making them ideal for weight management and overall health.

Part II: Foods to Avoid

Sugary Foods and Beverages

Here's a detailed, comprehensive content on "Sugary Foods and Beverages" related to a calorie diet food list, including sugary foods and beverages and why you should avoid them.

Each entry includes the sugary food or beverage, reason for avoidance, nutritional information, and serving size, all presented in a table format.

Sugary Food/Beverage	Reason to Avoid	Nutritional Information	Serving Size
Soda	High in added sugars and empty calories, can lead to weight gain, tooth decay, and increased risk of chronic diseases like	150 calories, 39g sugar, 0g protein, 0g fat per 12 oz can	12 oz can

Sugary Food/Beverage	Reason to Avoid	Nutritional Information	Serving Size
	diabetes and heart disease.		
Candy	High in added sugars and often high in unhealthy fats, providing little to no nutritional value, contributing to weight gain and tooth decay.	250 calories, 45g sugar, 1g protein, 9g fat per 2 oz serving	2 oz
Pastries	High in added sugars and unhealthy fats, leading to increased calorie intake and potential weight gain.	350 calories, 23g sugar, 5g protein, 17g fat per pastry	1 pastry

Sugary Food/Beverage	Reason to Avoid	Nutritional Information	Serving Size
	Often low in essential nutrients.		
Ice Cream	High in added sugars and saturated fats, leading to increased calorie intake and potential weight gain. Often low in essential nutrients.	210 calories, 20g sugar, 4g protein, 11g fat per 1/2 cup serving	1/2 cup
Sweetened Cereals	High in added sugars, can lead to spikes in blood sugar levels, and provide little nutritional value	120 calories, 12g sugar, 2g protein, 1g fat per 1 cup serving	1 cup

Sugary Food/Beverage	Reason to Avoid	Nutritional Information	Serving Size
	compared to whole grain or low-sugar cereals.		
Fruit Juice	Often contains added sugars and lacks the fiber of whole fruits, leading to rapid spikes in blood sugar levels.	110 calories, 24g sugar, 1g protein, 0g fat per 8 oz serving	8 oz
Energy Drinks	High in added sugars and often high in caffeine, can lead to weight gain, increased heart rate, and potential negative effects	160 calories, 38g sugar, 1g protein, 0g fat per 16 oz can	16 oz can

Sugary Food/Beverage	Reason to Avoid	Nutritional Information	Serving Size
	on heart health.		
Flavored Yogurt	Often contains high amounts of added sugars, reducing its nutritional value compared to plain yogurt.	150 calories, 19g sugar, 6g protein, 2g fat per 6 oz serving	6 oz
Chocolate Milk	High in added sugars, leading to increased calorie intake and potential weight gain.	208 calories, 24g sugar, 8g protein, 8g fat per 8 oz serving	8 oz
Cookies	High in added sugars and unhealthy fats, contributing to weight gain	160 calories, 14g sugar, 2g protein, 8g fat per 2 cookies	2 cookies

Sugary Food/Beverage	Reason to Avoid	Nutritional Information	Serving Size
	and potential health issues such as high cholesterol and diabetes.		
Cake	High in added sugars and unhealthy fats, leading to increased calorie intake and potential weight gain. Often low in essential nutrients.	250 calories, 30g sugar, 3g protein, 10g fat per slice	1 slice
Muffins	High in added sugars and unhealthy fats, contributing to increased calorie intake	400 calories, 37g sugar, 5g protein, 20g fat per muffin	1 muffin

Sugary Food/Beverage	Reason to Avoid	Nutritional Information	Serving Size
	and potential weight gain. Often low in essential nutrients.		
Sweetened Tea	Often contains high amounts of added sugars, leading to increased calorie intake and potential weight gain.	90 calories, 23g sugar, 0g protein, 0g fat per 8 oz serving	8 oz
Flavored Coffee Drinks	High in added sugars and unhealthy fats, leading to increased calorie intake and potential weight gain.	250 calories, 35g sugar, 2g protein, 8g fat per 12 oz serving	12 oz

Sugary Food/Beverage	Reason to Avoid	Nutritional Information	Serving Size
Granola Bars	Often contain high amounts of added sugars and can be high in unhealthy fats, despite being marketed as a healthy snack.	150 calories, 12g sugar, 3g protein, 5g fat per bar	1 bar

Summary:

This table provides a comprehensive guide to sugary foods and beverages to avoid when following a calorie-conscious diet. Each entry includes the sugary food or beverage, reasons to avoid it, nutritional information, and serving size.

Consuming high-sugar foods and drinks can lead to various health issues, including weight gain, tooth decay, and an increased risk of chronic diseases like diabetes and heart disease.

By avoiding these high-sugar items, you can better manage your calorie intake and improve your overall health.

Refined Carbohydrates

Here's a detailed, comprehensive content on "Refined Carbohydrates" related to a calorie diet food list.

This includes examples of refined carbohydrates and reasons why they should be avoided, presented in a table format.

Refined Carbohydrate	Description	Reasons to Avoid
White Bread	Made from refined flour, often stripped of fiber and nutrients.	High glycemic index, spikes blood sugar levels, low in fiber, can lead to weight gain and increased hunger.
White Rice	Processed to remove bran and germ, reducing fiber and nutrient content.	High in calories, low in fiber, can cause rapid blood sugar spikes, lacks essential nutrients compared to whole grains.
Pastries	Includes items like donuts, muffins, and croissants,	High in sugar and unhealthy fats, calorie-dense, can lead to weight gain and

Refined Carbohydrate	Description	Reasons to Avoid
	made with refined flour and sugar.	increased risk of heart disease and diabetes.
Sugary Cereals	Breakfast cereals high in added sugars and refined grains.	High in added sugars, low in fiber, can cause blood sugar spikes and crashes, contributes to poor nutrition and weight gain.
White Pasta	Made from refined wheat flour, lacks fiber and essential nutrients.	High glycemic index, low in fiber, can cause rapid increases in blood sugar levels, leading to hunger and overeating.
Cookies	Typically made with refined flour and high in added sugars and unhealthy fats.	High in sugar and calories, low in nutrients, can lead to weight gain, increased risk of chronic diseases like diabetes and heart disease.

Refined Carbohydrate	Description	Reasons to Avoid
Crackers	Often made with refined flour and contain added sugars and unhealthy fats.	Low in fiber and nutrients, high in calories, can contribute to weight gain and poor blood sugar control.
White Tortillas	Made from refined flour, lacking fiber and nutrients found in whole grain versions.	High glycemic index, can spike blood sugar levels, low in nutritional value, can contribute to weight gain.
Cakes	Made with refined flour, sugar, and often high in unhealthy fats.	Calorie-dense, high in sugars and unhealthy fats, can lead to weight gain, poor blood sugar control, and increased risk of chronic diseases.
Sweetened Beverages	Includes soda, energy drinks, and sweetened teas,	High in empty calories, can cause rapid spikes in blood sugar,

Refined Carbohydrate	Description	Reasons to Avoid
	high in added sugars.	contribute to weight gain, and increase the risk of diabetes and heart disease.
Candy	High in refined sugars and often contain unhealthy fats and additives.	Empty calories, high in sugars, can lead to weight gain, tooth decay, and increased risk of metabolic diseases.
Instant Noodles	Made from refined flour and often high in sodium and unhealthy fats.	Low in nutritional value, high in calories and sodium, can contribute to poor diet quality and health issues like hypertension.
Bagels	Made from refined flour, often large in	High in calories, low in fiber, can cause blood sugar spikes, and

Refined Carbohydrate	Description	Reasons to Avoid
	portion size and calorie-dense.	contribute to weight gain.
Pretzels	Typically made from refined flour and can be high in sodium.	Low in fiber and nutrients, high in sodium, can lead to overeating and poor blood sugar control.
Ice Cream	Often high in added sugars, unhealthy fats, and calories.	Calorie-dense, high in sugars and unhealthy fats, can lead to weight gain, poor blood sugar control, and increased risk of chronic diseases.

Summary:

Refined carbohydrates are foods that have been processed to remove their natural fiber and nutrients, resulting in a product that is often high in calories but low in essential nutrients.

Examples include white bread, white rice, pastries, sugary cereals, white pasta, cookies, crackers, white tortillas, cakes, sweetened beverages, candy, instant noodles, bagels, pretzels, and ice cream.

Reasons to Avoid Refined Carbohydrates:

1. **High Glycemic Index**: Refined carbs often have a high glycemic index, causing rapid spikes in blood sugar levels followed by crashes, which can lead to increased hunger and overeating.

2. **Low in Fiber**: The processing removes most of the fiber, which is essential for healthy digestion, blood sugar control, and satiety.

3. **Nutrient-Poor**: Refining strips away essential nutrients, making these foods calorie-dense but nutrient-poor.

4. **Weight Gain**: High-calorie content combined with low satiety can contribute to weight gain and obesity.

5. **Increased Risk of Chronic Diseases**: Consuming refined carbs regularly is linked to a higher risk of chronic conditions like type 2 diabetes, heart disease, and metabolic syndrome.

For a healthier diet, it's recommended to focus on whole grains, fruits, vegetables, and other nutrient-dense foods that provide sustained energy and support overall health.

Processed and Packaged Foods

Here's a detailed, comprehensive content on "Processed and Packaged Foods" related to a calorie diet food list. The table includes various processed and packaged foods, reasons to avoid them, and pertinent information.

Food	Why You Should Avoid It	Calories	Other Nutritional Concerns
Soda	High in added sugars and empty calories, leading to weight gain and increased risk of diabetes and heart disease.	150 calories per 12 oz can	High sugar (39g), no nutrients
Potato Chips	High in calories, unhealthy fats, and sodium, contributing to weight gain and heart health issues.	152 calories per 1 oz (15 chips)	High fat (10g), high sodium (170mg)

Food	Why You Should Avoid It	Calories	Other Nutritional Concerns
Candy Bars	Loaded with sugars and unhealthy fats, providing empty calories with little to no nutritional value.	250-280 calories per bar	High sugar (24g), high fat (14g)
Instant Noodles	High in sodium, unhealthy fats, and often contain preservatives and artificial flavors.	380 calories per package	High sodium (1,760mg), low protein (7g)
Frozen Pizzas	High in calories, unhealthy fats, and sodium, often made with refined flours and preservatives.	300-400 calories per slice	High sodium (700-900mg), high fat (18g)

Food	Why You Should Avoid It	Calories	Other Nutritional Concerns
Packaged Baked Goods	High in added sugars, unhealthy fats, and often contain preservatives and artificial ingredients.	200-500 calories per serving	High sugar (20-35g), high fat (12-25g)
Processed Meats	High in sodium, unhealthy fats, and often contain nitrates and preservatives linked to cancer risk.	150-300 calories per serving	High sodium (800-1,200mg), high fat (15-25g)
Breakfast Cereals	Often high in added sugars and low in fiber, leading to blood sugar spikes and lack of satiety.	110-150 calories per serving	High sugar (10-20g), low fiber (1-2g)

Food	Why You Should Avoid It	Calories	Other Nutritional Concerns
Microwave Popcorn	Can be high in unhealthy fats and sodium, often contains artificial flavors and preservatives.	120-150 calories per cup	High sodium (250-300mg), high fat (10g)
Ice Cream	High in sugars and unhealthy fats, leading to excess calorie intake and weight gain.	200-300 calories per 1/2 cup	High sugar (20-25g), high fat (12-20g)
Energy Drinks	High in added sugars and caffeine, leading to energy crashes and potential heart issues.	110-160 calories per 8.4 oz can	High sugar (27-30g), high caffeine (80-100mg)

Food	Why You Should Avoid It	Calories	Other Nutritional Concerns
Packaged Granola Bars	Often high in added sugars and unhealthy fats, providing little nutritional value compared to whole food alternatives.	150-250 calories per bar	High sugar (10-15g), high fat (7-10g)
Canned Soups	High in sodium and often contain preservatives, leading to high blood pressure and other health issues.	150-200 calories per serving	High sodium (800-1,000mg), low fiber (2-3g)
Packaged Snack Cakes	High in added sugars, unhealthy fats, and artificial ingredients, contributing to	250-350 calories per serving	High sugar (25-35g), high fat (15-20g)

Food	Why You Should Avoid It	Calories	Other Nutritional Concerns
	poor nutrition and weight gain.		
Flavored Yogurts	High in added sugars, often contain artificial flavors and preservatives, less nutritious than plain yogurt with added fruit.	150-200 calories per container	High sugar (18-25g), low protein (5-7g)

Summary:

This table provides a detailed overview of processed and packaged foods that should be avoided in a calorie-conscious diet.

Each food entry includes the reasons for avoidance, calorie content, and other nutritional concerns.

Processed and packaged foods are typically high in added sugars, unhealthy fats, and sodium while offering little nutritional value.

They often contain preservatives and artificial ingredients that can contribute to various health issues, including weight gain, heart disease, diabetes, and high blood pressure.

Opting for whole, unprocessed foods is a healthier choice for maintaining a balanced and nutritious diet.

High Fat and Fried Foods

Here's a detailed, comprehensive content on "High Fat and Fried Foods" related to a calorie diet food list, including why these foods should be avoided.

The table includes the food, description, and reasons to avoid it.

Food	Description	Reasons to Avoid
French Fries	Deep-fried potato sticks typically high in salt and fat.	High in calories, trans fats, and sodium, leading to weight gain, increased cholesterol levels, and higher risk of heart disease.
Fried Chicken	Chicken pieces coated in batter and deep-fried.	High in calories, saturated fats, and trans fats, which contribute to heart disease, obesity, and inflammation.
Potato Chips	Thin slices of potato fried until crispy.	High in calories, unhealthy fats, and sodium, which can lead to weight gain, high blood pressure, and increased risk of chronic diseases.
Doughnuts	Deep-fried dough typically	Extremely high in sugar, unhealthy fats,

Food	Description	Reasons to Avoid
	covered in sugar or filled with sweet fillings.	and calories, contributing to obesity, diabetes, and cardiovascular problems.
Cheeseburgers	Ground beef patties with cheese, often fried and served with a bun.	High in saturated fats, cholesterol, and calories, which can lead to heart disease, obesity, and other metabolic disorders.
Fried Fish	Fish fillets coated in batter and deep-fried.	High in calories and unhealthy fats, which can negate the health benefits of the fish, leading to weight gain and heart problems.
Mozzarella Sticks	Cheese sticks breaded and deep-fried.	High in saturated fats, cholesterol, and calories, which contribute to heart disease, obesity, and

Food	Description	Reasons to Avoid
		increased cholesterol levels.
Onion Rings	Sliced onions coated in batter and deep-fried.	High in calories, unhealthy fats, and sodium, leading to weight gain, high blood pressure, and increased risk of cardiovascular diseases.
Fried Calamari	Breaded and deep-fried squid rings.	High in calories, unhealthy fats, and sodium, which can lead to weight gain, high cholesterol, and heart disease.
Egg Rolls	Deep-fried rolls filled with meat and vegetables.	High in calories, unhealthy fats, and sodium, contributing to weight gain, high blood pressure, and increased risk of chronic diseases.

Food	Description	Reasons to Avoid
Fried Rice	Rice stir-fried with oil, often with added meats and vegetables.	High in calories, unhealthy fats, and sodium, which can lead to weight gain, high blood pressure, and increased risk of cardiovascular diseases.
Buffalo Wings	Chicken wings deep-fried and coated in spicy sauce.	High in calories, saturated fats, and sodium, contributing to weight gain, high cholesterol, and heart disease.
Pizza (High-fat Toppings)	Pizza topped with high-fat meats like pepperoni, sausage, and extra cheese.	High in saturated fats, calories, and sodium, leading to weight gain, high cholesterol, and increased risk of cardiovascular diseases.
Quesadillas	Flour tortillas filled with cheese	High in saturated fats, calories, and sodium, which can contribute to weight gain, high

Food	Description	Reasons to Avoid
	and sometimes meat, then fried.	cholesterol, and heart disease.
Churros	Deep-fried dough pastries, often sprinkled with sugar or filled with sweet fillings.	Extremely high in sugar, unhealthy fats, and calories, leading to obesity, diabetes, and cardiovascular problems.

Summary:

This table highlights various high-fat and fried foods that should be avoided in a calorie-conscious diet. These foods, ranging from French fries and fried chicken to doughnuts and mozzarella sticks, are typically high in unhealthy fats, calories, and sodium.

Consuming these foods regularly can lead to weight gain, high cholesterol, heart disease, diabetes, and other chronic health issues. For a healthier diet, it's advisable to opt for baked, grilled, or steamed alternatives that are lower in unhealthy fats and calories.

High Calorie Condiments and Sauces

Here's a detailed, comprehensive content on "High-Calorie Condiments and Sauces" related to a calorie diet food list.

This table includes high-calorie condiments and sauces, their nutritional information, serving size, and reasons why they should be avoided on a calorie-conscious diet.

Condiment/Sauce	Nutritional Information (per serving)	Serving Size	Reason to Avoid
Mayonnaise	94 calories, 0g protein, 10g fat, 1g carbs	1 tablespoon	High in unhealthy fats and calories, contributing to weight gain. Often used in large quantities, making it easy to consume excessive calories without realizing it.
Ranch Dressing	129 calories, 1g protein, 13.4g fat, 2.1g carbs	2 tablespoons	High in calories and fats, often containing

Condiment/Sauce	Nutritional Information (per serving)	Serving Size	Reason to Avoid
			added sugars and preservatives. Commonly overused in salads, leading to calorie-dense meals.
Ketchup	20 calories, 0g protein, 0g fat, 5g carbs	1 tablespoon	Contains added sugars, contributing to unnecessary calorie intake. Often used liberally, which can quickly add

Condiment/Sauce	Nutritional Information (per serving)	Serving Size	Reason to Avoid
			up in calories.
Barbecue Sauce	70 calories, 0g protein, 0g fat, 18g carbs	2 tablespoons	High in added sugars and calories. Frequent use can lead to consuming large amounts of hidden sugars, contributing to weight gain and potential blood sugar spikes.

Condiment/Sauce	Nutritional Information (per serving)	Serving Size	Reason to Avoid
Honey Mustard	60 calories, 0g protein, 4g fat, 7g carbs	1 tablespoon	Contains added sugars and fats. While it can add flavor, the calorie count can quickly add up, especially in larger servings.
Thousand Island	114 calories, 0.2g protein, 10.2g fat, 7.6g carbs	2 tablespoons	High in calories, fats, and sugars. Often used in large quantities in salads, making

Condiment/Sauce	Nutritional Information (per serving)	Serving Size	Reason to Avoid
			healthy meals calorie-dense.
Tartar Sauce	70 calories, 0g protein, 7g fat, 2g carbs	2 tablespoons	High in fats and calories. Typically paired with fried foods, compounding calorie intake.
Peanut Butter	188 calories, 8g protein, 16g fat, 6g carbs	2 tablespoons	Though nutritious, it's calorie-dense and easy to overeat. High in fats, which can quickly add up in calories when consumed in

Condiment/Sauce	Nutritional Information (per serving)	Serving Size	Reason to Avoid
			large amounts.
Sour Cream	60 calories, 1g protein, 5g fat, 1g carbs	2 tablespoons	High in fats and calories. Frequently used as a topping, which can lead to excessive calorie intake without adding significant nutritional value.
Pesto Sauce	80 calories, 1g protein, 8g fat, 1g carbs	1 tablespoon	High in fats and calories due to ingredients

Condiment/Sauce	Nutritional Information (per serving)	Serving Size	Reason to Avoid
			like olive oil and nuts. While healthy in moderation, can easily lead to excessive calorie intake in larger portions.
Cheese Sauce	70 calories, 3g protein, 5g fat, 3g carbs	2 tablespoons	High in fats and calories, often used in large quantities. Contains added preservatives and can

Condiment/Sauce	Nutritional Information (per serving)	Serving Size	Reason to Avoid
			significantly increase the calorie content of a dish.
Gravy	50 calories, 1g protein, 3g fat, 5g carbs	1/4 cup	High in fats and often made with added butter or drippings from meats. Can quickly increase the calorie content of meals, especially in larger servings.

Condiment/Sauce	Nutritional Information (per serving)	Serving Size	Reason to Avoid
Syrup (Maple or Pancake)	52 calories, 0g protein, 0g fat, 13g carbs	1 tablespoon	High in sugars and calories. Commonly used in large amounts on breakfast foods, leading to significant calorie intake from added sugars.
Chocolate Syrup	50 calories, 0g protein, 0g fat, 13g carbs	1 tablespoon	High in sugars and calories. Often used as a topping or mix-in, which can

Condiment/Sauce	Nutritional Information (per serving)	Serving Size	Reason to Avoid
			add unnecessary calories and sugars to otherwise healthy foods.
Hollandaise Sauce	67 calories, 0.5g protein, 7.2g fat, 0.5g carbs	1 tablespoon	High in fats and calories. Typically used in breakfast dishes like eggs Benedict, adding significant calories and fats to meals that could

Condiment/Sauce	Nutritional Information (per serving)	Serving Size	Reason to Avoid
			otherwise be lighter.

Summary:

This table provides a comprehensive guide to high-calorie condiments and sauces that should be avoided on a calorie-conscious diet.

These condiments and sauces, such as mayonnaise, ranch dressing, and barbecue sauce, are high in calories, fats, and sugars. They can easily lead to excessive calorie intake, especially when used in large quantities, which is common. Avoiding or limiting these high-calorie additions can help in maintaining a balanced, lower-calorie diet, supporting weight loss and overall health.

Part III: Meal Planning and Recipes

Creating Balanced Meals

Creating balanced meals is essential for maintaining a healthy diet, especially when following a calorie-conscious plan. A balanced meal typically includes a variety of food groups, such as lean proteins, whole grains, fruits, vegetables, and healthy fats.

Incorporating these elements ensures that you receive the necessary nutrients while managing your calorie intake. For example, a balanced lunch might include a grilled chicken breast, a serving of quinoa, a side salad with a variety of colorful vegetables, and a small portion of avocado.

This combination provides protein, fiber, vitamins, minerals, and healthy fats, all within a controlled calorie limit.

Planning meals in advance can help you stay on track with your dietary goals.

Start by selecting a variety of lean proteins like chicken, fish, tofu, and legumes. Pair these with whole grains such as brown rice, quinoa, or whole wheat pasta.

Adding a generous portion of vegetables not only boosts the nutrient content but also helps you feel fuller with fewer calories. Fruits can serve as a natural dessert, offering sweetness and essential vitamins without the added sugars found in processed treats.

Additionally, including healthy fats like olive oil, nuts, and seeds can improve satiety and provide important nutrients.

Recipes can be tailored to fit within your calorie goals while still being delicious and satisfying. For breakfast, consider a vegetable omelet made with egg whites and a side of whole grain toast.

This meal is high in protein and fiber, keeping you full throughout the morning.

For lunch, a quinoa salad with mixed greens, cherry tomatoes, cucumbers, and a light vinaigrette dressing can be both refreshing and nutritious.

Dinner could include baked salmon with a side of roasted sweet potatoes and steamed broccoli, offering a well-rounded mix of protein, healthy fats, and complex carbohydrates.

Portion control is crucial when creating balanced meals. Even healthy foods can contribute to weight gain if consumed in excessive amounts. Using smaller plates, measuring serving sizes, and being mindful of portion sizes can help you manage your calorie intake more effectively.

For instance, a serving of lean protein should be about the size of a deck of cards, while a serving of cooked grains should be roughly the size of a tennis ball. Vegetables can be consumed in larger portions, filling half of your plate to ensure you get plenty of fiber and nutrients.

Meal prep can save time and ensure you have healthy options readily available. Spend a few hours each week preparing meals and snacks.

Cook large batches of grains and proteins that can be used throughout the week, chop vegetables for quick salads or stir-fries, and portion out snacks like nuts and fruit.

Having pre-prepared meals can reduce the temptation to grab fast food or unhealthy snacks when you're short on time. It also allows for better portion control and adherence to your calorie goals.

Balancing meals also involves paying attention to the nutritional quality of the foods you choose. Opt for whole, minimally processed foods over refined and packaged items.

Whole foods tend to be lower in added sugars, unhealthy fats, and sodium, making them better for overall health and weight management.

Additionally, incorporating a variety of foods ensures you get a wide range of nutrients, supporting different bodily functions and promoting overall well-being.

Lastly, it's important to enjoy your meals and find satisfaction in healthy eating. Experiment with different recipes, flavors, and cooking methods to keep your meals interesting and enjoyable.

Remember that a balanced diet is not about deprivation but about making smarter choices that nourish your body and support your health goals.

Building a Low-calorie Plate

Creating balanced meals is essential for maintaining a healthy diet, especially when following a calorie-conscious plan. A balanced meal typically includes a variety of food groups, such as lean proteins, whole grains, fruits, vegetables, and healthy fats.

Incorporating these elements ensures that you receive the necessary nutrients while managing your calorie intake. For example, a balanced lunch might include a grilled chicken breast, a serving of quinoa, a side salad with a variety of colorful vegetables, and a small portion of avocado.

This combination provides protein, fiber, vitamins, minerals, and healthy fats, all within a controlled calorie limit.

Planning meals in advance can help you stay on track with your dietary goals. Start by selecting a variety of lean proteins like chicken, fish, tofu, and legumes.

Pair these with whole grains such as brown rice, quinoa, or whole wheat pasta. Adding a generous portion of vegetables not only boosts the nutrient content but also helps you feel fuller with fewer calories.

Fruits can serve as a natural dessert, offering sweetness and essential vitamins without the added sugars found in processed treats. Additionally, including healthy fats like olive oil, nuts, and seeds can improve satiety and provide important nutrients.

Recipes can be tailored to fit within your calorie goals while still being delicious and satisfying. For breakfast, consider a vegetable omelet made with egg whites and a side of whole grain toast. This meal is high in protein and fiber, keeping you full throughout the morning.

For lunch, a quinoa salad with mixed greens, cherry tomatoes, cucumbers, and a light vinaigrette dressing can be both refreshing and nutritious. Dinner could include baked salmon with a side of roasted sweet potatoes and steamed broccoli, offering a well-rounded mix of protein, healthy fats, and complex carbohydrates.

Portion control is crucial when creating balanced meals. Even healthy foods can contribute to weight gain if consumed in excessive amounts. Using smaller plates, measuring serving sizes, and being mindful of portion sizes can help you manage your calorie intake more effectively.

For instance, a serving of lean protein should be about the size of a deck of cards, while a serving of cooked grains should be roughly the size of a tennis ball. Vegetables can be consumed in larger portions, filling half of your plate to ensure you get plenty of fiber and nutrients.

Meal prep can save time and ensure you have healthy options readily available. Spend a few hours each week preparing meals and snacks. Cook large batches of grains and proteins that can be used throughout the week, chop vegetables for quick salads or stir-fries, and portion out snacks like nuts and fruit.

Having pre-prepared meals can reduce the temptation to grab fast food or unhealthy snacks when you're short on time. It also allows for better portion control and adherence to your calorie goals.

Balancing meals also involves paying attention to the nutritional quality of the foods you choose. Opt for whole, minimally processed foods over refined and packaged items. Whole foods tend to be lower in added sugars, unhealthy fats, and sodium, making them better for overall health and weight management.

Additionally, incorporating a variety of foods ensures you get a wide range of nutrients, supporting different bodily functions and promoting overall well-being.

Lastly, it's important to enjoy your meals and find satisfaction in healthy eating. Experiment with different recipes, flavors, and cooking methods to keep your meals interesting and enjoyable.

Remember that a balanced diet is not about deprivation but about making smarter choices that nourish your body and support your health goals. By creating balanced meals that are both nutritious and satisfying, you can maintain a healthy weight and improve your overall quality of life.

Portion Control Tips

Portion control is an essential aspect of maintaining a calorie-conscious diet, and it plays a significant role in meal planning and recipe creation. By focusing on the amount of food consumed in each meal, individuals can manage their calorie intake more effectively and support their weight management goals.

One of the most effective ways to implement portion control is by using smaller plates, bowls, and utensils. This simple trick can help reduce the amount of food eaten by making portions appear larger, thereby promoting a feeling of fullness and satisfaction with less food.

Understanding proper portion sizes is crucial. For instance, a serving of lean protein, such as chicken or fish, should be about the size of a deck of cards or the palm of your hand.

Carbohydrates like rice or pasta should be limited to about the size of a tennis ball. Incorporating more vegetables into your meals can help you feel fuller without adding many calories. Vegetables are low in calories but high in volume, allowing you to eat larger portions of these foods while still keeping your calorie intake in check.

When meal planning, it is beneficial to pre-portion snacks and meals. By preparing individual servings of snacks like nuts, fruits, or yogurt in advance, you can avoid the temptation to overeat from larger packages.

Similarly, cooking meals in bulk and dividing them into single-serving containers can make it easier to control portions and ensure that you have balanced, calorie-conscious meals ready to go throughout the week. This approach also saves time and reduces the likelihood of reaching for less healthy options when you're in a hurry.

Mindful eating practices can also support portion control. Taking the time to eat slowly and savor each bite can help you recognize your body's hunger and fullness cues. This awareness can prevent overeating and promote better digestion.

Additionally, avoiding distractions such as television or smartphones during meals allows you to focus on the food and the eating experience, further enhancing your ability to control portions.

Using portion control tools such as measuring cups, food scales, and portion control plates can provide a visual guide to appropriate serving sizes.

These tools can help you become more familiar with what a healthy portion looks like and can aid in adjusting your eating habits over time. They are especially useful when trying new recipes or when you're unsure about the correct portion size for a particular food.

Incorporating high-fiber foods into your meals is another effective strategy for portion control. Foods rich in fiber, such as whole grains, legumes, fruits, and vegetables, can help you feel fuller for longer periods.

This satiety can reduce the likelihood of overeating and can support your overall calorie management efforts. Additionally, staying hydrated is important as thirst is often mistaken for hunger. Drinking water before and during meals can help you feel full and reduce the amount of food consumed.

Portion control does not mean you have to eliminate your favorite foods. It's about enjoying them in moderation.
By balancing indulgent foods with healthier options and being mindful of portion sizes, you can still enjoy a varied and satisfying diet.

Planning for occasional treats and incorporating them into your overall meal plan can help you stay on track with your calorie goals without feeling deprived. This balanced approach fosters a healthier relationship with food and supports long-term adherence to your dietary goals.

Sample Meal Plans

Sample meal plans for a calorie-conscious diet can help structure balanced and nutritious meals throughout the day. Starting with breakfast, a well-rounded option could be a bowl of Greek yogurt topped with fresh blueberries and a sprinkle of granola.

Greek yogurt provides a substantial amount of protein to keep you feeling full, while blueberries add natural sweetness and antioxidants. A small amount of granola adds crunch without overwhelming the calorie count. Pairing this with a glass of water or green tea can help keep you hydrated and refreshed for the day ahead.

For mid-morning snacks, consider having a handful of almonds or a small apple. Almonds offer healthy fats and protein, which are essential for sustained energy levels.

An apple provides fiber and natural sugars, making it a great option to curb any mid-morning hunger pangs. These snacks are easy to carry and can be enjoyed on the go, ensuring you stay on track with your calorie goals without sacrificing nutrition.

Lunch could consist of a mixed green salad with grilled chicken breast, cherry tomatoes, cucumber, and a light vinaigrette. The grilled chicken adds lean protein to your meal, while the fresh vegetables contribute vitamins and minerals.

A light vinaigrette, made with olive oil and vinegar, provides healthy fats and flavor without adding excessive calories. This meal is not only filling but also refreshing, perfect for a midday break.

In the afternoon, a snack of baby carrots with hummus can be both satisfying and nutritious. Baby carrots are low in calories but high in fiber and vitamins.

Hummus, made from chickpeas, offers protein and healthy fats, making it a balanced snack option. This combination is not only tasty but also easy to prepare and pack, ensuring you have a healthy option readily available.

Dinner could feature a serving of baked salmon with a side of quinoa and steamed broccoli. Salmon is a rich source of omega-3 fatty acids and high-quality protein.

Quinoa is a versatile grain that provides essential amino acids and complements the protein in salmon.
Steamed broccoli adds fiber, vitamins, and minerals, making this meal nutrient-dense and satisfying. Baking the salmon with a drizzle

of olive oil, lemon juice, and herbs ensures a flavorful yet low-calorie dish.

For an evening snack or dessert, consider a small bowl of mixed berries or a piece of dark chocolate. Mixed berries, such as strawberries, raspberries, and blackberries, are low in calories and high in antioxidants.

They can satisfy your sweet tooth without leading to a significant calorie intake. A piece of dark chocolate, in moderation, can also be a delightful treat. It provides antioxidants and can be a perfect way to end your day on a sweet note.

Staying hydrated throughout the day is crucial, so incorporating water, herbal teas, or sparkling water with meals and snacks can help.

Avoid sugary drinks and opt for beverages that support hydration without adding unnecessary calories.

7Day Low-calorie Meal Plan

Creating a 7-day low-calorie meal plan involves thoughtful selection of nutrient-dense foods to ensure you meet your nutritional needs while maintaining a calorie deficit.

Start the week with a breakfast of Greek yogurt topped with fresh berries and a sprinkle of granola, providing a balanced mix of protein, fiber, and antioxidants.

For lunch, a hearty salad with mixed greens, grilled chicken breast, cherry tomatoes, cucumbers, and a light vinaigrette keeps you full without adding too many calories.

Dinner can be a grilled salmon fillet with a side of steamed broccoli and quinoa, offering a rich source of omega-3 fatty acids, vitamins, and complex carbohydrates.

On the second day, a breakfast smoothie made with spinach, a banana, almond milk, and a scoop of protein powder starts your day on a nutritious note.

A vegetable stir-fry with tofu, bell peppers, snap peas, and carrots in a light soy sauce makes for a satisfying lunch.

Dinner might include a baked turkey breast served with roasted Brussels sprouts and sweet potato wedges, providing a balance of lean protein, fiber, and essential vitamins.

Mid-week, opt for oatmeal cooked with water, topped with sliced almonds and a dash of cinnamon for breakfast. A quinoa salad with black beans, corn, avocado, and a lime-cilantro dressing offers a refreshing and filling lunch.

Dinner can feature a lean beef stir-fry with a variety of colorful vegetables like bell peppers, broccoli, and mushrooms served over brown rice, ensuring a nutritious and low-calorie meal.

For the fourth day, start with a breakfast of scrambled egg whites with spinach and tomatoes. A chickpea and vegetable stew, made with tomatoes, zucchini, and onions, served with a small portion of whole grain bread, makes a delicious and fiber-rich lunch.

Dinner can be grilled shrimp skewers with a side of mixed vegetables and a small serving of couscous, providing a light yet filling meal rich in protein and nutrients.

On the fifth day, enjoy a breakfast parfait with layers of low-fat yogurt, mixed berries, and a sprinkle of chia seeds.

A whole grain wrap filled with grilled chicken, mixed greens, and a light mustard dressing makes a convenient and low-calorie lunch. For dinner, a bowl of lentil soup with a side of steamed green beans and a slice of whole grain bread offers a hearty and nutritious end to the day.

For the weekend, start Saturday with a vegetable omelet made with egg whites, bell peppers, onions, and a touch of low-fat cheese. A large bowl of mixed greens with grilled salmon, cherry tomatoes, cucumber, and a lemon vinaigrette provides a light and satisfying lunch.

Dinner can be a roasted chicken thigh with a side of sautéed kale and a small serving of brown rice, ensuring a balanced meal that is both low in calories and rich in nutrients.

Finish the week with a breakfast of whole grain toast topped with avocado and a poached egg.

A Mediterranean salad with mixed greens, feta cheese, olives, cherry tomatoes, and a balsamic dressing makes for a flavorful and nutritious lunch.

For dinner, enjoy a bowl of vegetable and barley soup with a side of roasted carrots, ensuring you close the week with a meal that is both filling and healthy while maintaining your low-calorie diet goals.

Vegetarian and Vegan Options

When planning a calorie-conscious diet, vegetarian and vegan options can play a crucial role in ensuring variety and nutritional balance. These diets emphasize plant-based foods, which are often lower in calories and higher in essential nutrients.

Incorporating a range of vegetables, fruits, legumes, nuts, seeds, and whole grains can provide the necessary vitamins, minerals, and antioxidants while keeping calorie intake in check. A key aspect of meal planning is to ensure that meals are both satisfying and nutritionally complete, providing adequate protein, healthy fats, and complex carbohydrates.

One way to achieve a balanced vegetarian meal is by focusing on protein-rich plant foods such as beans, lentils, chickpeas, tofu, and tempeh.

For example, a chickpea and vegetable stir-fry can be a flavorful and filling option, offering protein from the chickpeas and a variety of vitamins from the mixed vegetables.

Similarly, a lentil soup, enriched with spices and herbs, can provide a hearty and warming meal that's low in calories but high in fiber and protein, aiding in satiety and digestive health.

To enhance the nutritional profile of vegan meals, incorporating a variety of colorful vegetables is essential. A rainbow salad with spinach, bell peppers, tomatoes, carrots, and red cabbage not only looks appealing but also provides a wide array of nutrients and antioxidants.

Adding a dressing made from tahini, lemon juice, and garlic can increase the healthy fat content, making the salad more satiating. Another option is to prepare a quinoa and black bean bowl, topped with avocado, corn, and a squeeze of lime, delivering a balance of protein, fiber, and healthy fats.

Breakfast options for vegetarians and vegans can be diverse and nutritious as well. Overnight oats made with almond milk, chia seeds, and fresh berries can be a quick and easy option that is both satisfying and nutrient-dense.

Another excellent breakfast choice is a smoothie bowl, blended with spinach, banana, and plant-based protein powder, and topped with granola, nuts, and seeds.

These options not only provide essential vitamins and minerals but also keep the calorie count in check while ensuring a good start to the day.

Snacks are an important part of any diet plan, and vegetarian and vegan diets offer a plethora of healthy options. Fresh fruit, such as apples or berries, paired with a handful of nuts, can be a convenient and nutritious snack.

Hummus with carrot sticks or whole-grain crackers is another excellent choice, offering a good balance of protein, fiber, and healthy fats. For a more indulgent treat, dark chocolate with almonds or a homemade energy bar made from dates, oats, and peanut butter can satisfy cravings while still being relatively low in calories.

For lunch and dinner, a variety of hearty yet low-calorie dishes can be prepared. A vegetable curry with a coconut milk base, served over brown rice or quinoa, can be both flavorful and nutritious. Similarly, a vegan chili made with black beans, tomatoes, and spices can provide a protein-packed meal that is rich in fiber and low in calories.

Grilled vegetable skewers with a side of couscous or a baked sweet potato stuffed with a mixture of beans, corn, and avocado can offer a delicious and satisfying meal without excessive calories.

Incorporating these vegetarian and vegan options into a calorie-conscious diet can be both enjoyable and beneficial. By focusing on a variety of plant-based foods, one can achieve a balanced and nutritious diet that supports overall health and well-being while keeping calorie intake under control.

This approach not only promotes a healthier lifestyle but also introduces a wide array of flavors and textures to meals, making the dietary journey enjoyable and sustainable.

Healthy Recipe Ideas

Breakfast

Smoothie bowls are a delicious and nutritious way to start the day, especially when keeping an eye on calorie intake. For a tropical smoothie bowl, blend together one frozen banana, one cup of frozen mango chunks, one cup of spinach, and half a cup of unsweetened almond milk.

Pour the thick smoothie into a bowl and top with fresh kiwi slices, a tablespoon of chia seeds, and a handful of granola. This combination provides approximately 250 calories, 5 grams of protein, 4 grams of fat, and 50 grams of carbohydrates per serving. The preparation time is around 10 minutes, making it a quick and easy breakfast option.

Another variation is a berry smoothie bowl, which is both refreshing and packed with antioxidants. Blend one cup of frozen mixed berries, half a frozen banana, and half a cup of unsweetened almond milk until smooth.

Pour into a bowl and top with fresh strawberries, a tablespoon of hemp seeds, and a few coconut flakes.

This bowl contains about 200 calories, 3 grams of protein, 3 grams of fat, and 40 grams of carbohydrates per serving. The preparation time for this bowl is also approximately 10 minutes, making it a convenient and healthy start to the day.

Oatmeal with fresh fruit is another excellent breakfast option for those following a calorie-conscious diet. For a classic oatmeal recipe, combine half a cup of rolled oats with one cup of water or unsweetened almond milk in a saucepan.

Bring to a boil, then reduce heat and simmer for 5-7 minutes, stirring occasionally. Once the oats are cooked, top with half a sliced banana, a handful of fresh blueberries, and a sprinkle of cinnamon. This serving provides around 150 calories, 4 grams of protein, 2.5 grams of fat, and 27 grams of carbohydrates.

Cooking time is approximately 10 minutes, making it a quick and wholesome breakfast choice.

For a more indulgent twist, try an apple cinnamon oatmeal. Start by cooking half a cup of rolled oats with one cup of water or unsweetened almond milk.

In a separate pan, sauté one chopped apple with a teaspoon of coconut oil and a dash of cinnamon until tender. Stir the cooked apple into the oatmeal and top with a tablespoon of chopped walnuts.

This hearty breakfast offers approximately 200 calories, 5 grams of protein, 6 grams of fat, and 33 grams of carbohydrates. The total cooking time is around 15 minutes, providing a warm and satisfying meal to kickstart the day.

A nutritious and versatile oatmeal option is the berry almond oatmeal. Prepare half a cup of rolled oats with one cup of water or unsweetened almond milk.

Once cooked, stir in a handful of fresh raspberries and blueberries, and top with a tablespoon of sliced almonds. This combination delivers roughly 180 calories, 5 grams of protein, 5 grams of fat, and 30 grams of carbohydrates.

The preparation and cooking time are about 10 minutes, making it a quick and balanced breakfast choice.

For those who prefer overnight oats, they are a convenient and time-saving breakfast option.

Combine half a cup of rolled oats with one cup of unsweetened almond milk, a tablespoon of chia seeds, and half a teaspoon of vanilla extract in a jar.

Stir well, cover, and refrigerate overnight. In the morning, top with fresh strawberries and a drizzle of honey. This overnight oat recipe provides about 200 calories, 6 grams of protein, 7 grams of fat, and 30 grams of carbohydrates.

The preparation time is just 5 minutes, with no cooking required, making it perfect for busy mornings.

Another tasty overnight oat variation is the chocolate banana overnight oats. Mix half a cup of rolled oats with one cup of unsweetened almond milk, a tablespoon of cocoa powder, a tablespoon of chia seeds, and half a mashed banana in a jar.

Refrigerate overnight and top with banana slices and a sprinkle of dark chocolate chips in the morning. This recipe offers around 250 calories, 6 grams of protein, 8 grams of fat, and 40 grams of carbohydrates.

The preparation time is also just 5 minutes, providing a quick and delicious start to the day without the need for cooking.

Lunch

Quinoa Salad with Veggies is a nutritious and delicious option for a calorie-conscious lunch.

For this recipe, you'll need the following ingredients: 1 cup quinoa, 2 cups water, 1 cup cherry tomatoes (halved), 1 cucumber (diced), 1 bell pepper (diced), 1/4 cup red onion (finely chopped), 1/4 cup fresh parsley (chopped), 1/4 cup feta cheese (crumbled), 2 tablespoons olive oil, 1 tablespoon lemon juice, salt, and pepper to taste.

To prepare the quinoa salad, start by rinsing the quinoa under cold water. In a medium saucepan, bring the quinoa and water to a boil. Reduce the heat to low, cover, and simmer for 15 minutes or until the water is absorbed and the quinoa is tender. Remove from heat and let it cool.

In a large bowl, combine the cherry tomatoes, cucumber, bell pepper, red onion, parsley, and feta cheese. Add the cooled quinoa and mix well. In a small bowl, whisk together the olive oil, lemon juice, salt, and pepper. Pour the dressing over the salad and toss to combine.

Nutritional information per serving includes 250 calories, 8g protein, 12g fat, 28g carbohydrates, and 4g fiber. The serving size is approximately 1 cup, and the total cooking time is about 25 minutes. This quinoa salad is a perfect balance of protein, healthy fats, and fiber, making it a satisfying and nutritious lunch option.

Grilled Chicken Wrap is another excellent choice for a healthy lunch. The ingredients required for this recipe are: 1 boneless, skinless chicken breast, 1 tablespoon olive oil, salt, pepper, 1/2 teaspoon paprika, 1/2 teaspoon garlic powder, 1 whole wheat tortilla, 1/2 avocado (sliced), 1/2 cup lettuce (shredded), 1/4 cup tomatoes (diced), and 2 tablespoons Greek yogurt.

To prepare the grilled chicken wrap, start by preheating the grill to medium-high heat. In a small bowl, mix the olive oil, salt, pepper, paprika, and garlic powder. Brush the chicken breast with the seasoned oil mixture. Grill the chicken for 6-7 minutes per side or until the internal temperature reaches 165°F.

Remove the chicken from the grill and let it rest for a few minutes before slicing it into strips. Warm the whole wheat tortilla in a dry skillet over medium heat for about 1 minute on each side. Lay the tortilla flat and spread the Greek yogurt in the center. Add the sliced chicken, avocado, lettuce, and tomatoes. Roll up the tortilla, tucking in the sides as you go.

Nutritional information per serving includes 350 calories, 30g protein, 15g fat, 25g carbohydrates, and 7g fiber. The serving size is 1 wrap, and the total cooking time is approximately 20 minutes. This grilled chicken wrap is packed with protein and healthy fats, making it a filling and nutritious lunch option.

Both of these lunch recipes are designed to be low in calories while providing essential nutrients to keep you satisfied and energized throughout the day. The quinoa salad with veggies offers a refreshing and light option, while the grilled chicken wrap provides a heartier and more substantial meal.

By incorporating these recipes into your lunch rotation, you can enjoy delicious and healthy meals that align with your calorie-conscious diet goals.

Dinner

Baked Salmon with Asparagus

Ingredients:

4 salmon fillets (4 oz each), 1 lb asparagus, 2 tbsp olive oil, 1 lemon (sliced), 2 cloves garlic (minced), salt and pepper to taste, 1 tsp dried dill.

Instructions:

Preheat the oven to 400°F. Arrange salmon fillets on one side of a baking sheet and asparagus on the other side. Drizzle olive oil over both the salmon and asparagus. Sprinkle garlic, salt, pepper, and dill over the salmon and asparagus.

Place lemon slices on top of the salmon. Bake for 12-15 minutes until the salmon is opaque and flakes easily with a fork, and the asparagus is tender.

Nutritional Information:

Per serving: 290 calories, 25g protein, 18g fat, 5g carbs.

Serving Size:	Cooking Time:
1 salmon fillet and 1/4 lb asparagus.	12-15 minutes.

Stir-Fried Tofu with Vegetables

Ingredients:

1 block firm tofu (14 oz), 1 red bell pepper (sliced), 1 yellow bell pepper (sliced), 1 cup broccoli florets, 2 tbsp soy sauce, 1 tbsp sesame oil, 2 cloves garlic (minced), 1 tbsp ginger (minced), 1 tbsp sesame seeds, 1 green onion (sliced).

Instructions:

Press the tofu to remove excess water, then cut into cubes. Heat sesame oil in a large skillet over medium-high heat. Add tofu cubes and cook until golden brown, about 5-7 minutes. Remove tofu from skillet and set aside. In the same skillet, add garlic and ginger, sauté for 1 minute.

Add bell peppers and broccoli, stir-fry for 5-7 minutes until tender-crisp. Return tofu to the skillet, add soy sauce, and stir well. Sprinkle with sesame seeds and green onion before serving.

Nutritional Information: Per serving: 250 calories, 14g protein, 15g fat, 15g carbs.

Serving Size:	Cooking Time:
1 cup.	12-15 minutes.

Hummus with Veggie Sticks

Ingredients:

1 can chickpeas (15 oz, drained and rinsed), 1/4 cup tahini, 2 tbsp olive oil, 1 lemon (juiced), 2 cloves garlic, 1/2 tsp cumin, salt to taste, 1/4 cup water, 1 cucumber (sliced), 2 carrots (sliced), 1 bell pepper (sliced).

Instructions:

In a food processor, combine chickpeas, tahini, olive oil, lemon juice, garlic, cumin, and salt. Process until smooth, adding water as needed to achieve desired consistency. Serve hummus with sliced cucumber, carrots, and bell pepper.

Nutritional Information:

Per serving: 180 calories, 5g protein, 10g fat, 15g carbs.

Serving Size:

1/4 cup hummus with veggie sticks.

Cooking Time:
10 minutes.

Greek Yogurt with Berries

Ingredients:

1 cup Greek yogurt, 1/2 cup mixed berries (blueberries, strawberries, raspberries), 1 tbsp honey, 1 tbsp chia seeds.

Instructions:

In a bowl, combine Greek yogurt and honey. Top with mixed berries and chia seeds.

Nutritional Information:

Per serving: 150 calories, 10g protein, 3g fat, 20g carbs.

Serving Size: 1 cup.

Cooking Time: 5 minutes.

These recipes provide a variety of options that are both nutritious and calorie-conscious, making them suitable for those looking to maintain a healthy diet. Each dish includes a balance of proteins, fats, and carbohydrates to ensure a well-rounded meal that supports overall health and wellness goals.

Conclusion

Adopting a calorie-conscious diet can be an effective strategy for weight management and overall health improvement. By carefully selecting foods that are nutrient-dense and low in empty calories, you can create a balanced diet that supports your wellness goals.

Focusing on whole, unprocessed foods such as vegetables, fruits, lean proteins, and whole grains ensures that you receive essential nutrients while maintaining a controlled calorie intake. This approach not only aids in weight loss but also enhances energy levels and overall vitality.

Incorporating a variety of foods into your diet is crucial to prevent nutritional deficiencies and maintain interest in your meals. A diet rich in colorful vegetables and fruits provides vitamins, minerals, and antioxidants that support bodily functions and protect against diseases.

Lean proteins from sources like chicken, fish, beans, and tofu help build and repair tissues, while whole grains supply sustained energy and fiber for digestive health. By diversifying your food choices, you ensure a broad spectrum of nutrients that contribute to overall well-being.

Portion control is another key element in a calorie-conscious diet. Even healthy foods can contribute to weight gain if consumed in large quantities. Paying attention to serving sizes and listening to your body's hunger cues can help you avoid overeating.

Mindful eating practices, such as eating slowly and savoring each bite, can enhance your awareness of fullness and satisfaction, reducing the likelihood of consuming excess calories.

Hydration plays a significant role in a calorie-conscious diet. Drinking plenty of water throughout the day supports metabolic processes, aids digestion, and can help control appetite.

Sometimes, thirst is mistaken for hunger, leading to unnecessary calorie consumption. Incorporating water-rich foods like cucumbers, watermelon, and leafy greens can also contribute to your hydration needs while providing essential nutrients.

High-calorie condiments and sauces can easily sabotage a calorie-conscious diet. These items often contain hidden sugars, unhealthy fats, and unnecessary calories.

Being mindful of these additions and opting for healthier alternatives, such as fresh herbs, spices, and homemade dressings, can make a significant difference. Reading labels and understanding the nutritional content of condiments can help you make informed choices that align with your dietary goals.

Vegetarian and vegan options can be excellent choices for a calorie-conscious diet, offering a range of nutrient-dense foods that are typically lower in calories than animal-based products.

Plant-based diets emphasize whole grains, legumes, fruits, and vegetables, which are high in fiber and essential nutrients while being low in unhealthy fats and calories.

These diets can be both satisfying and beneficial for weight management and overall health, promoting a balanced intake of macronutrients and micronutrients.

Consistency and planning are essential for the success of a calorie-conscious diet. Preparing meals in advance and having healthy snacks on hand can help you stay on track and resist the temptation of high-calorie, unhealthy options.

Tracking your food intake using apps or journals can provide insight into your eating patterns and help you make adjustments as needed.

By staying committed to your dietary goals and making informed food choices, you can achieve and maintain a healthy weight while enjoying a varied and satisfying diet.

www.ingramcontent.com/pod-product-compliance
Lightning Source LLC
Chambersburg PA
CBHW050101230526
45470CB00004B/1623